Health Policy Developments

Issue 3

Reinhard Busse, Sophia Schlette (eds.)

Health Policy Developments

Issue 3:
Focus on Accountability,
(De)Centralization,
Information Technologies

| **Verlag** Bertelsmann**Stiftung**

Bibliographic information published by Die Deutsche Bibliothek

Die Deutsche Bibliothek lists this publication in the
Deutsche Nationalbibliografie; detailed bibliographic data
is available on the Internet at http://dnb.ddb.de.

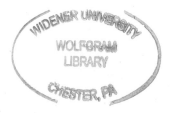

© 2004 Verlag Bertelsmann Stiftung, Gütersloh
Responsible: Sophia Schlette
Copy editor: Michael Kühlen
Production editor: Christiane Raffel
Cover design: Nadine Humann
Cover illustration: Aperto AG, Berlin
Typesetting: digitron GmbH, Bielefeld
Print: Hans Kock Buch- und Offsetdruck GmbH, Bielefeld
ISBN 3-89204-796-0

www.bertelsmann-stiftung.de/publications

Contents

Editorial

The Bertelsmann Stiftung has a tradition of comparative policy research and international benchmarking. In Germany, it has established a reputation for providing advice and innovative problem-solving in the field of economic and social politics.

The International Reform Monitor (www.reformmonitor.org), initiated in 1999 and now in its sixth year, is one example of this benchmark expertise. It primarily covers social and labor market issues. An example of the Foundation's expertise in comparative health policy research is "Reformen im Gesundheitswesen" (Esche, Böcken and Butzlaff (eds.) 2000), a study that compared health policy reforms in eight countries.

The success of both projects underscored the need and the potential demand for timely and regular information on health policy issues in countries with similar socioeconomic patterns. To this end, the Foundation established a separate monitoring tool, the International Network Health Policy and Reform.

The International Network Health Policy and Reform

Since 2002, the International Network has brought together health policy experts from 16 countries from around the world to report on current health reform issues and health policy developments in their countries. Geared toward implementation, the Network aims to narrow the gap between research and policy, providing timely information on what works and what does not in health policy reform. Participating countries were chosen from a German perspective; we specifically looked for countries with relevant reform experience to enrich the debate in this country.

Partner institutions were selected taking into account their expertise in health policy and management, health economics or public health. Our network is interdisciplinary; our experts are economists, political scientists, physicians or lawyers. Many of them have considerable experience as policy advisers, others in international comparative research.

Australia	Centre for Health Economics, Research and Evaluation (CHERE), University of Technology, Sydney
Austria	Institute for Advanced Studies, Vienna
Canada	Canadian Policy Research Networks (CPRN), Ottawa
Denmark	Institute of Public Health, Health Economics, University of Southern Denmark, Odense
Finland	STAKES, National Research and Development Center for Welfare and Health, Helsinki
France	CREDES, Centre de Recherche d'Etude et de Documentation en Economie de la Santé, Paris
Germany	Bertelsmann Stiftung, Gütersloh Department Health Care Management, Berlin University of Technology (TUB)
Japan	National Institute of Population and Social Security Research (IPSS), Tokyo
Netherlands	Institute of Health Policy and Management (iBMG), Erasmus University Rotterdam
New Zealand	Centre for Health Services, Research and Policy, University of Auckland
Republic of Korea	Seoul National University
Singapore	Department of Community, Occupational & Family Medicine, National University of Singapore (NUS)
Spain	Research Centre for Economy and Health (Centre de Reserca en Econimia i Salut, CRES), University Pompeu Fabra, Barcelona
Switzerland	Until 2003: Centre for Economic Sciences, University of Basel From 2004: Università della Svizzera Italiana, Lugano
UK	LSE Health & Social Care, London School of Economics and Political Science (LSE)

USA	The Commonwealth Fund, New York
	Institute for Global Health (IGH), University of California Berkeley/San Francisco

Survey preparation and proceedings

Issues for reporting were determined jointly based on what the network partners identified as the most pressing issues for reform. Subsequently, the issues were arranged into clusters:
- Sustainable financing of health care systems (funding and pooling of funds, remuneration and paying providers)
- Human resources
- Quality issues
- Benefit basket and priority setting
- Access
- Responsiveness and empowerment of patients
- Political context, decentralization and public administration
- Health system organization/integration across sectors
- Long-term care
- Role of private sector
- New technology
- Pharmaceutical policy
- Prevention
- Public health

If an issue did not fit into one of the clusters, participants could create an additional category to report the topic.

Reporting criteria

For each survey, partner institutes select up to five health policy issues according to the following criteria:
- Relevance and scope
- Impact on status quo
- Degree of innovation (measured against national and international standards)
- Media coverage/Public attention

For each issue, partner institutions fill out a questionnaire aimed at describing and analyzing the dynamics or processes of the idea or policy under review. At the end of the questionnaire, our correspondents give their opinion regarding the expected outcome of the reported policy. Finally, they also rate the policy in terms of system dependency/transferability of a reform approach.

The process stage of a health policy development is illustrated with an arrow showing the phase(s) a reform is in. A policy or idea does not necessarily have to evolve step by step. Also, depending on the dynamics of discussion in a given situation, a health policy issue may well pass through several stages during the time observed:

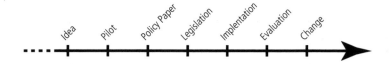

Idea refers to new and newly raised approaches voiced or discussed in different fora. Idea could also mean "early stage": any idea floating but not anywhere near formal inception. That way, a "stock of health policy ideas in development" is established, permitting the observation of ideas appearing and disappearing through time and "space."

Pilot characterizes any innovation or model experiment implemented at a local or institutional level.

Policy Paper means any formal written statement or policy paper short of a draft bill. Included under this heading is also a growing degree of acceptance of an idea within a relevant professional community.

Legislation covers all steps of the legislative process from the formal introduction of a bill/draft piece of legislation to parliamentary hearings, driving forces, the influence of professional lobbyists in the process and the effective enactment or rejection of the proposal.

Implementation: This stage is about all measures taken towards legal and professional implementation and adoption of a policy. Implementation does not necessarily result from legislation; it may also follow the evidence of best practice tried out in model or pilot projects.

Evaluation refers to all health policy issues scrutinized for their impact during the period observed. Any review mechanism, internal or external, mid-term or final, is reported under this heading.

Change may be a result of evaluation or abandonment of development.

Policy ratings

A second figure is used to give the reader an indication of the character of the policy. For this purpose, three criteria are shown: public visibility, impact and transferability.

Public Visibility refers to the public awareness and discussion of the reform, as demonstrated by media coverage or public hearings. The ratings range from "very low" (on the left) to "very high" (on the right).

Impact: Ranging from "marginal" (on the left) to "fundamental" (on the right), this rating criterion illustrates the structural or systemic scope and relevance of a reform given the country's current health care system.

Transferability: This rating indicates whether a reform approach could be adapted to other health care systems. Our experts assess the degree to which a policy or reform is strongly context-dependent (on the left) to neutral with regard to a specific system, i.e., transferable (on the right).

The figure below illustrates a policy that scores low on visibility and impact but average on transferability.

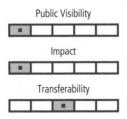

Project management

The Bertelsmann Stiftung's Health Program organizes and implements the half-yearly surveys. The Department of Health Care Management, Berlin University of Technology (TUB), assisted with the development of the semi-standardized questionnaire (see Appendix). We owe special thanks to Susanne Weinbrenner, who produced the draft for this summarizing report, to Celia Bohannon for doing an excellent proof-reading job, as well as to Christina Brickenkamp and Heike Clostermeyer in the Bertelsmann Stiftung for managerial and editorial support.

The results from the third biannual survey, covering the period November 2003 to April 2004, are presented in this booklet. Out of 67 reported reforms, 31 were selected.

While we describe current developments from the reporting period in detail on our Web site, we chose a somewhat different approach to present the findings in this report. Criteria for selection were scope, continuity and presence in public debate during and beyond the reporting period proper. With this in mind, we looked at topics from the first and the second survey independently of their present stage of development or implementation.

Reports from the first, second and third survey rounds can be looked up and researched at www.healthpolicymonitor.org, the Network's Web site. Both the detailed description on the Web and this brochure draw upon the partner institutions' reports and do not necessarily reflect the Bertelsmann Stiftung's point of view.

Thanks of course go to all experts from our partner institutions:

Tetsuya Aman, Rob Anderson, Michael O. Appel, Toni Ashton, Mickael Bech, Mette Birk-Olsen, Iva Bolgiani, Wim Buiten, David Cantarero Prieto, David Casado, Karine Chevreul, Terkel Christiansen, Agnès Couffinhal, Luca Crivelli, J. K. (Han) van Dijk, Gianfranco Domenighetti, Massimo Filippini, Michel Grignon, Tom van der Grinten, Marion Haas, Jane Hall, Jan-Kees Helderman, Maria M. Hofmarcher, Noboyuki Izumida, Ilmo Keskimäki, Wendy van der Kraan, Soonman Kwon, Meng Kin Lim, Anita Lee, Véronique Lucas, Esther Martínez García, Lisa Maslove, Carol Medlin, Hennamari Mikkola, Kjeld Møller Pedersen, Florence Naudin, Valérie Paris, Anniek Peelen, Dominique Polton, Jaume Puig i Junoy, Gerda Raas, Monika Riedel, Mary Ries, Ray Robinson, Gerald Röhrling, Masayo Sato, Elizabeth Savage, Catherine Sermet, Pieter Vos, Lauri Vuorenkoski, Karen Wallstadt, Sarah Weston, and Karen White.

Comments and suggestions on the third half-yearly report are more than welcome and can be addressed to the editors. This series will continue to evolve, change, and, as we hope, improve. That is why any input will be helpful.

Reinhard Busse
Sophia Schlette

Introduction

The third issue of "Health Policy Developments" pays special attention to five concurrent health policy topics, all of them high on health policy agendas in a variety of developed countries:

- Accountability and participation
- Coordination of care
- Public health and prevention
- Centralization versus decentralization
- Technical innovations and bioethics

Two of these topics, accountability and prevention, are of particular interest to the Bertelsmann Stiftung.

As an independent yet not neutral player in the German health care system, the Foundation examines health care services and health policy reform from the specific, usually underrepresented viewpoint of the insured themselves. Much lip service has been paid to the importance of the informed patient, the patient as the focus of attention, and the patient's responsibility to participate in the maintenance of good health and in the treatment process. In practice, however, little has changed. Many stakeholders—insurers, physicians, politicians, and the health care industry—claim to know what is best for the patients or so-called health care consumers.

Accountability and participation

Behind these claims often lurk profit interests, professional self-esteem, or—a variation of profit interests—the politician's pursuit of re-election. While this is not the place to challenge the legitimacy of business or power interests, recent experience has indeed shown just how important patient views are to policymakers. In fact, politicians are increasingly sensitive and attentive to their voters' concerns about health care.

The reports described in this chapter shed light on promising attempts to foster patient participation and individual responsibility in an independent, unbiased way.

Numerous international publications have indicated the importance of citizens and patients participating in the process of health care delivery, as well as in the planning and implementation of health care reforms.

For example, the European health ministers convened by the WHO in Ljubljana in 1996 stated in the Ljubljana Charter in 1996: "Health care reforms must address citizens' needs taking into account, through the democratic process, their expectations about health and health care. They should ensure that the citizen's voice and choice decisively influence the way in which health services are designed and operate. Citizens must also share responsibility for their own health." (www.euro.who.int/eprise/main/WHO/AboutWHO/Policy/20010927_5)

Within this arena, the culture of health care provision is changing in response to concerns about the safety and quality of the services provided, resource constraints and an increasingly educated and informed population, forcing governments to ensure that care is provided efficiently and effectively.

People are no longer content to be treated as passive recipients of what others decide is good for them. They want to be involved in the planning, management and delivery of health care services; they want to ensure that the care they receive is safe, effective and appropriate to their needs. Particularly with regard to chronic diseases, participation in prevention and treatment is crucial to optimize outcomes. Therefore, individuals should actively participate throughout the health care process—from the promotion of health and well-being to the management of disease.

Coordination of care　The number of people with one or multiple chronic conditions is increasing. These people typically receive care from different sectors of the social system and often from different providers within a sector. This makes health care delivery complex and confusing, and often inefficient as well.

Health Policy Developments (HPD) 1/2003 already reported on the issue of integrated care—one of the organizational changes within health care systems regarded as having a high potential for both cost containment and quality improvement.

The term "coordination of care" is often used interchangeably with case management, care management, disease management, and integrated care. Several variations of care coordination have been developed to improve care, promote independence and reduce unnecessary use of health services (see case studies from Australia, Canada, France, Germany and the United Kingdom). The coordination occurs along a continuum from social to medical care in a range of settings.

Prevention is another priority in the Bertelsmann Stiftung's health program activities. The Foundation sees prevention as a key policy tool to increase efficiency in the health care system, control costs in the long run and increase economic growth by generating employment in the new branches of an expanding wellness and health service industry.

Public health and prevention

In Germany, prevention rose higher on the health agenda after 2000, when an advisory council to the Federal Ministry of Health estimated that prevention could well reduce total health care costs by 25 to 30 percent. Currently, prevention accounts for only 4.5 percent of total health expenditures (see table on p. 36). Attempts to pay more attention to an area with prospectively high returns on investment have generally been hampered by the short-term attitude of most players. Why invest if future gains are likely to be harvested by others in charge, at a much later point in time and under a different government?

Efforts to curb pressure on labor costs and re-boost economic growth in Germany have much to do with the way social insurance funds generate their revenues from salaries and incomes. If preventive measures can effectively keep health care costs and premiums in check, cost containment gains strength as a political argument for promoting (and investing in) prevention.

Long-term rationale

While the majority of stakeholders display general goodwill towards prevention as a priority, there can be little doubt that criticism would erupt if funding were shifted from curative to preventive care. Such a reform would certainly bring standard delivery procedures under scrutiny; if pursued wholeheartedly, it would turn the system upside down. It would also produce new winners and losers, forcing traditional stakeholders to adjust. To increase overall acceptance of such a paradigm shift, the Ministry of Health and Social Security seeks to underpin its prevention goals

Paradigm shift toward prevention

with scientific evidence showing a positive return on investment —evidence that is emerging elsewhere and abroad.

Prevention and the economic context

It is general knowledge that health care systems face increasing budget strains. In this regard, public health measures and prevention are coming to the fore.

Concerning the delivery of care, gains have been made in a number of areas, most notably within acute care. But many challenges remain, for example in the prevention and management of chronic diseases. Furthermore, the future will bring new tasks, such as overcoming the epidemic of obesity and nutrition-related diseases.

Good health depends on high-quality and effective health care systems as well as on the social and environmental context. Thus, public health and prevention measures focus on setting the conditions for a healthy life. The major determinants of health offer great potential for reducing the burden of disease and promoting the health of the general population. These can be categorized as personal behavior and lifestyles; community influences that can promote or damage health; living and working conditions; access to health services; and general socioeconomic, cultural and environmental conditions.

Decentralization versus ...

In many countries, federal systems and subsidiary organizations for health services delivery and other social services are well-established. In Europe, the Nordic countries have a long tradition of decentralization in some types of health care systems as well as social health insurance systems. More recently, Mediterranean countries such as Italy and Spain have decentralized their political systems, including health care. Within these countries or systems, local responsibility and accountability are seen as effective tools promoting reasonable use of scarce health care resources.

... (Re-) Centralization

However, a reverse development can be observed as well. The trend goes toward strengthening midlevel administration and/or reinforcing the normative and control functions of central health authorities or the ministry of health. Denmark, Finland, Spain and Switzerland report reforms aimed at modifying or amending the existing structures of territorial decision-making. Examples from these countries (partly covered in previous HPD issues) show that policies must always be reassessed against the particular background of a specific policy issue. Also, the balance between centralizing and decentralizing competencies needs continuing adjustments.

Advances in technical as well as biological sciences are clearly influencing health, health care and society as a whole.

Concerning information technologies (IT), Health Policy Developments (HPD) 2/2003 focused on issues of data security. HPD 3/2004 now reports on Web-based innovation of IT solutions aimed at enhancing the quality of information as well as improving the exchange of data. In addition, these technologies have the potential to enhance consumer autonomy.

Technical innovations and bioethics

Bioethics is a very delicate matter. Surveys from France and Singapore report on this highly contentious issue. In line with the adoption of European Union legislation and with pressure to update a 1994 law, France is debating a revision of the legislative framework on bioethics. Issues such as organ transplantation, medically assisted reproduction, therapeutic cloning and gene patenting are all on the lawmakers' agenda. During the intense and lengthy debate, the approach changed from a rather liberal to a rigid conservative one. Singapore, in contrast, merely amended its transplantation act to counter the shortage in organ donations.

Finally, in line with the Health Policy Network's news and monitoring function, the last chapter follows up on developments reported in Issue 1/2003 or 2/2003, particularly on expanding health care coverage to uninsured citizens in the United States and on the further development of rejected reform proposals such as the second revision of the health insurance act in Switzerland and the new organizational framework of sickness insurance in France.

Newsflash

Accountability and Participation

Health care systems and health care providers are increasingly held accountable to deliver services in a user-friendly, effective and efficient way. Many countries are responding to this demand. Reports from Denmark and England describe quite comprehensive plans to enhance accountability and participation within a range of services.

Canada has established a Health Council to report to the public and give independent advice on reforms. Unfortunately, the Council's competencies have already been trimmed compared to the original idea. Germany introduced a patient representative within the scope of the Social Health Insurance Modernization Act.

Finland and the Netherlands are piloting different forms of personal budgets in certain areas of their health care systems. These vouchers allow patients individual choice of services and providers.

England: Choice and responsiveness in the English National Health Service

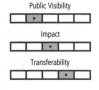

Public Visibility

Impact

Transferability

Offering more choice is an important objective of public sector reform in England. Based on the NHS (National Health Service) Plan published in 2002, the aims of extending user choice were outlined in the December 2003 report "Building on the Best: Choice, Responsiveness and Equity in the NHS."

Following this report, the British government recently announced a policy on choice and responsiveness that will be built into the new planning framework for the NHS.

Specific elements of this policy are:

- *Virtual health space:* Starting next year, patients will have access to a secure personal health organizer ("health space") on the Internet, where information will be recorded and where they will be able to register preferences as a means of facilitating better shared decision-making.
- *Better access to primary care:* Steps to improve access to primary care include providing more and varied capacity, extending the existing telephone advice line, expanding walk-in clinics, offering more nurse-led clinics, and expanding independent sector treatment centers.
- *Hospital treatment—choice of time and place:* A national pilot program launched in July 2002 offers more choice to patients who have waited over six months for heart surgery. The government intends to offer these extended choices to all patients waiting for surgery by August 2004, and by December 2005 it plans to offer all patients who require surgery the choice among four to five hospitals.

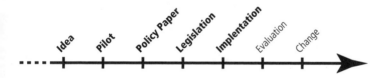

These plans are to be implemented by top-down performance management; that is, expectations are built into performance targets, supported by the so-called Modernisation Agency, although the plans include financial incentives for hospital performance.

As this policy is the result of a national consultation exercise, it is quite consensual. Criticism is limited to the perceived trade-off between equity and choice. The National Audit Office is planning a review of the various policies on choice.

Sources and further reading:
Secretary of State for Health. Building on the best: Choice, responsiveness and equity in the NHS. (Cm 6079) The

Stationery Office, London 2003. www.dh.gov.uk/asset-Root/04/06/84/00/04068400.pdf.

Denmark: An open and transparent health care system

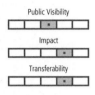

Public Visibility

Impact

Transferability

Quality indicators for patient orientation

In December 2003, the Danish government published a discussion paper on an open and transparent health care system. A follow-up to the paper "Strategy for the health care system—the patient first," it details the quality indicators announced earlier.

The government paper states several objectives and instruments. The primary objective is to improve the quality of treatment. Secondly, the Minister of Health plans to enable patients to make informed choices concerning their treatment, such as choosing a particular hospital. To attain these goals, stronger incentives for better performance (e.g., a "money follows patient" scheme) will be implemented. Increasing competition is seen as an effective way of promoting quality. More information, better information and easier access to information are regarded as prerequisites for informed choice.

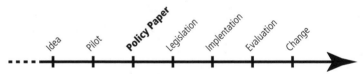

Overall, the plan may be viewed as an attempt of the Liberal Danish government to introduce more market-oriented incentives and greater consumer orientation. However, as the Minister of Health, who initiated the paper, has very little or no support from other stakeholders (such as the Minister of Finance, the counties or the hospitals), the outcome remains uncertain.

Sources and further reading:
Indenrigs- og Sundhetsministeriet: www.im.dk (mostly in Danish)

Canada: Independent health policy advice

In December 2003, the Health Council of Canada was established. The original idea—piloted in Saskatchewan and subsequently in other provinces such as Alberta, Ontario and Que-
bec—was to establish a quality council independent of the government, made up of representatives of the public, providers,
health policy experts and governments. The main objective was to
create a source of non-politicized and comprehensive advice on
health care reforms.

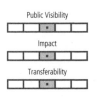

In contrast to the original idea, which was to provide advice
and recommendations on health care reforms, the Council's
mandate has been limited to monitoring and reporting on the
implementation of policies in the Health Care Renewal Accord.
Furthermore, the idea of an independent council has been wea-
kened. Half of the current council members are government
representatives.

**Reporting rather
than advising**

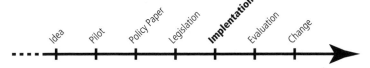

It remains to be seen whether the Council will achieve its potential for enhanced public accountability. This will depend on the
resources dedicated to the Council and its ability to identify and
report independently on the issues that most concern the Canadian population.

Sources and further reading:
First Ministers' Accord on Health Renewal: www.hc-sc.gc.
ca/english/hca2003/accord.html
Commission on the Future of Health Care in Canada.
Building on Values: The Future of Health Care in Canada.
Final Report of the Romanow Commission. November
2002. www.hc-sc.gc.ca/english/pdf/romanow/pdfs/HCC_
Final_Report.pdf.

Finland: Vouchers in social and health care

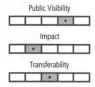

A law adopted early in 2004 provides the legal framework for the general use of vouchers in social and health services, particularly in home care services. Voucher projects in child day care had been piloted through the nineties.

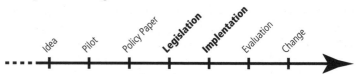

Vouchers may serve a variety of purposes. They are viewed as an alternative instrument to finance and provide social and health services. From the consumers' point of view, they may increase a client's freedom of choice and help elderly people to stay at home. From an economic perspective, vouchers may have a potential to increase cost-effectiveness of services, stimulate an expansion of the supply of services and create jobs by encouraging small firms to enter home care markets.

In Finland, vouchers are tax-free fixed sums granted by municipalities for eligible clients. A municipal officer determines eligibility, offering the voucher as an alternative to municipal services. However, there is no right to claim a voucher.

The value of the voucher is influenced by the client's income and deductible, which is not allowed to exceed the municipality's user charge.

Extended choice— extended costs? The reform is based on international experiences, mainly from Sweden, national pilot projects and a survey of various professional experts and institutions. However, the service voucher system is expected to increase the cost of home care services by about €31 million (or six percent) per year. It was widely debated in the media and was one of the social policy issues in the March

2003 elections. Nonetheless, there is no noteworthy controversy on this issue.

Sources and further reading:

Heikkilä, Matti, Sinikka Törmä and Kati Mattila. A service voucher in child day care, a report on the national pilot project. Ministry of Social Affairs and Health, National Research and Development Centre for Welfare and Health: Stakes Reports 216/1997, Gummerus Oy, Jyväskylä 1997 (in Finnish with an English summary)

Mikkola, Hennamari. International experience of the use of service vouchers in social welfare and health care. Ministry of Social Affairs and Health 15/2003, Helsinki 2003 (in Finnish with an English summary).

Niemelä, Jutta. The use of service vouchers in the social and health service in different countries. Ministry of Social Affairs and Health 15/1997, Helsinki 1997.

Räty, Tarmo, Kalevi Luoma and Pasi Aronen. Service vouchers in municipal social services. Government Institute for Economic Research 325/2004, Helsinki 2004 (in Finnish with an English summary).

Vaarama, Marja, Sinikka Törmä, Seppo Laaksonen and Voutilainen Päivi. The report on the vouchers in the support of informal care, a pilot project. Ministry of Social Affairs and Health and National Research and Development Centre for Welfare and Health: Stakes Reports 10/1999, Helsinki 1999 (in Finnish with an English summary)

Netherlands: Client-linked personal budgets

Health care of the Dutch population is covered by the ZFW (Ziekenfondswet) on a benefit-in-kind basis; continuation of income (i.e., sick pay) is covered by the ZW (Ziektewet); and long-term care, as well as mental health care, is covered by the National Health Insurance Scheme under the Exceptional Medical Expenses Act (Algemene Wet Bijzondere Ziektekosten, AWBZ).

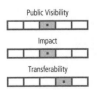

Public Visibility

Impact

Transferability

As part of the reform of the AWBZ, client-linked personal budgets were introduced in April 2003. Budget holders are now able to purchase care by themselves. The aim is to change the health care system from a supply-driven to a demand-driven system.

From supply to demand

The benefits under AWBZ are based on functional categories: household assistance, personal care, nursing care, activating assistance, medical care, hotel function and support assistance. Within these categories, medical care and long-term care in nursing homes are excluded from client-linked budgets (but short-term stays away from home are included).

An advisor from the Regional Indication Office (RIO) carries out a needs assessment to determine the budget level of each patient. Based on the assessment, a so-called gross budget is calculated. Depending on personal income and the kind of care needed, a personal contribution between 20 and 60 percent is deducted. The resulting net budget is transferred to the patient's personal bank account.

Entrepreneurs in individual health care

Budget holders are monitored by the Regional Care Offices (Zorgkantoor) through random checks. Spending of the official budget has to be recorded for at least 98.5 percent of the funds. To some degree, money can be spent for services other than the assessed needs.

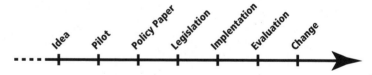

All in all, patients face quite a lot of administrative work. They must invite bids; negotiate services, prices and contracts; arrange for social insurance and taxes of their respective provider; and, finally, record all activities.

Backup is provided by a self-help organization called Per Saldo, as well as by the care administration office and the CLB Service Centre of the Social Insurance Bank.

Expectations are high and positive, but a previous similar experiment showed that many patients (about 55 percent) would prefer to stay in the old system.

Sources and further reading:
Modernizing AWBZ: www.opkopzorg.nl (in Dutch)
Per Saldo, an organization of personal budget holders: www.pgb.nl/showpage.php?pa=234 (in English)

Coordination of Care

Chronic diseases present an increasing challenge worldwide; therefore, coordination of care is a constant in health policy debate.

Reports from Australia describe a collaborative care program for primary care that sets a framework of change management to improve care delivery, with emphasis on the chronically ill. Concrete projects are the coordinated care trials aiming at an explicitly planned multidisciplinary approach. While the Australian reforms are in part borrowed from the United Kingdom, England is piloting disease management programs modeled on U.S. programs. As shortcomings with the treatment of chronically ill patients became more and more evident, Germany has also introduced disease management programs for certain chronic diseases. Last but not least, the Canadian province of Ontario seeks to improve primary care by focusing on an interdisciplinary approach to health promotion and wellness with respect to chronic diseases.

Australia: Primary care collaboratives

Public Visibility

Impact

Transferability

In 2003, the Commonwealth Government announced a Primary Care Collaborative Program, to be implemented between 2004 and 2006.

This program is a large-scale change management program to improve service delivery and meet national objectives and goals, especially concerning chronic and complex conditions.

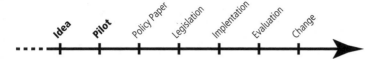

Experiences with the NHS Primary Care Collaborative in Great Britain and frustration with the inefficacy of traditional strategies to implement best practice in primary care have influenced this policy.

Australia seeking best practice

Terms and methodology are originally from the work of the Institute of Healthcare Improvement (IHI) in the US, which developed the collaborative method. Key features of this method are an expert reference panel, learning workshops followed by action periods, and finally tracing of changes.

There is no appreciable debate on this topic.

Sources and further reading:
Australian Primary Care Collaboratives Program: www. health.gov.au/pcd/programs/apccp/
Institute of Healthcare Improvement: www.ihi.org
National Primary Care Development Team: www.npdt.org

Australia: Coordinated care trials

Australia also aims to improve the management of chronic diseases by carrying out a series of coordinated care trials.

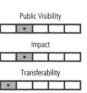

Currently, five second-round trials that started in late 2002 are underway. The results of the first round were somewhat disappointing, with no significant improvement of parameters (e.g., improved health and well-being). The second-round trials are using modified indicators. In addition, they run over a longer period and focus on minorities. The purpose of these trials is to test whether multidisciplinary explicit care planning and service coordination through pooling of funds for these purposes leads to improved health and well-being for people with chronic and complex conditions.

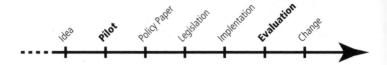

Idea   **Pilot**   Policy Paper   Legislation   Implementation   **Evaluation**   Change

Focusing on the marginalized

The trials focus on particular groups of the Australian population, such as Aborigines or Torres Strait Islanders. These groups have key health indicators comparable to those in developing countries but not to those of the average Australian population. The focus on ethnic minorities reflects a political and public health imperative to improve infrastructure and access to services as well as individual and community empowerment for this particular part of the population. Stakeholders are supportive, as they had already been involved before the first trial round. Concerns center chiefly on fund holding and the possibility of a loss of control over resource use.

Sources and further reading:
Commonwealth Department of Health and Ageing—Co-ordinated Care Trials: www.health.gov.au/hsdd/primcare/acoorcar/abtrials.htm
Commonwealth Department of Health and Ageing—Primary Care Initiatives: www.health.gov.au/hsdd/primcare/acoorcar/pubs/index.htm
Beilby, John, and Brita Pekarsky. Fundholding: learning from the past and looking to the future. *Medical Journal of Australia* (176) 6 2002: 321–325.
Commonwealth Department of Health and Aged Care. The Australian Coordinated Care Trials: Background and Trial Descriptions. 1999.
Esterman, Adrian J., and David I. Ben-Tovim. The Australian coordinated care trials: success or failure? *Medical Journal of Australia* (177) 9 2002: 469–470.

England: The management of chronic disease

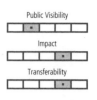

Public Visibility

Impact

Transferability

Under the leadership of the (soon to be abolished) NHS Modernization Agency, in England at present 18 Primary Care Trusts are piloting the Evercare approach of United Health Care, a U.S. health maintenance organization. Beyond that, the Secretary of State for Health announced in March 2004 that starting in 2004/ 2005, each of the 28 Strategic Health Authorities would establish case management for high-risk patients.

In the United Kingdom at large, an estimated one third of the population is suffering from chronic diseases. These patients account for 80 percent of general practitioners' consultations. Even though the general practitioner-system in the UK is regarded as working well, it is not performing satisfactorily with regard to integration and coordination of care for people with chronic conditions.

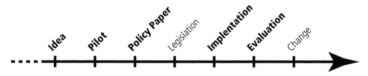

As data from the United States suggest considerably lower hospitalization rates within some managed care organizations, the English Department of Health and think tanks are giving higher priority to chronic disease management.

Testing new ways of care delivery

The case management tests are not a politically controversial issue but an example of advanced attempts to improve micromanagement of the health care system, driven by professionals.

Sources and further reading:
Department of Health 2004. A better life for people with chronic disease. Press release. March 11, 2004.
Dixon, Jennifer, Richard Lewis, Rebecca Rosen, Belinda Finlayson, and Diane Gray. Managing chronic disease: what can we learn from US experience. London: King's Fund, 2004.
Feachem, Richard et al. Getting more for their dollar: A

comparison of the NHS with California's Kaiser Permanente. British Medical Journal (324) 2002: 135–141.
NHS Confederation. Chronic Disease: The hidden agenda. London 2003.
Talbot-Smith, Alison, et al. Questioning the claims from Kaiser. British Journal of General Practice (54) 503 2004: 415–421.

Germany: Disease Management Programs combine quality and financial incentives

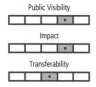

Public Visibility

Impact

Transferability

On February 27, 2003, the German Federal Insurance Office accredited the first Disease Management Programs (DMPs) for breast cancer. In April, the first DMPs for diabetes were accredited.

The German DMPs are the result of the Act to Reform the Risk-Structure Compensation (RSC) Scheme, which had been based on average expenditures by age and sex only. As chronically ill persons were not adequately taken into account, the competition among sickness funds for insured members concentrated on the healthy. The introduction of DMPs addressed this problem by building a new RSC category. The high level of activity by the sickness funds—as well as the fierce opposition from physicians—is a valid indicator that the incentives are working.

The Act defined a complicated process for the introduction of DMPs. The newly formed Coordinating Committee was charged with recommending to the ministry of health which major chronic diseases to select and the minimum common requirements for the respective DMPs. This was a new division of labor: The self-governing bodies propose, and the ministry passes an ordinance.

The Act also stipulated the factors the Coordinating Committee has to take into account when selecting a disease for DMPs, such as number of patients, potential for quality improvement and high expenditures. The Act then described the process: Based on the defined minimum requirements, sickness funds contract with providers and establish their own provisions for informing and convincing their members to subscribe (which is voluntary), educating patients and evaluating the programs.

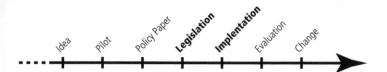

Such a DMP "package" then needs to be accredited by the Federal Insurance Office; only then may the sickness fund actually run the program. Just a few weeks after the bill became law, the Co-ordinating Committee proposed the first four conditions for DMPs: diabetes, breast cancer, asthma and coronary heart disease.

First DMPs for diabetes, breast cancer, asthma, CHD

A major blockade occurred in the summer of 2002, when a national assembly of all regional physicians' associations passed a motion that no regional association should sign a DMP contract. After the elections, progress was smoother but still full of hurdles before the first DMPs started in spring 2003.

While the actual long-term results of the DMPs will not be available for a few years, the first winners are the chronically ill, who are no longer seen as "bad risks" but as a customer group worth attracting and caring for.

> *Sources and further reading:*
> Busse, Reinhard: Disease Management Programs in Germany's Statutory Health Insurance System—A Gordian solution to the adverse selection of chronically ill in competitive markets? *Health Affairs* (23) 3 2004: 56–67.

Canada: Primary care reform

In Canada, primary care reform has been recommended for decades by several commissions, including two high-profile commissions.

In March 2001, the Ontario Family Health Network was created to implement primary care reform in the province.

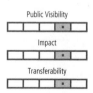

33

Combining prevention and primary care

At the moment, the majority of Canadian general practitioners and family physicians provide mostly curative or rehabilitative services. Under the new regime, patients will receive care from interdisciplinary teams focusing on wellness and health promotion. The reform will offer incentives to enhance comprehensive, coordinated care particularly for chronic diseases and focus on prevention.

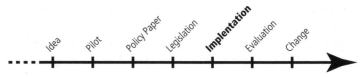

Ontario's primary care model

At the moment, the majority of Canadian General Practitioners and Family Physicians are providing mostly curative or rehabilitative services. To emphasize prevention and integration of care, Ontario recently introduced a new model, the Family Health Groups. These groups are designed to be a hybrid of the Family Health Networks created in March 2001, and traditional primary care services. When participating in a network model, physicians are largely paid on a capitation base. Under the new system, physicians are mostly paid individually on a fee-for-service basis with premiums and bonuses for preventive services. Nurse practitioners and new information technologies are funded through Family Health Groups as well.

The Ontario medical association has been involved in developing the models. Yet concerns remain about accountability when physicians are not the primary provider.

Coordination focusing on prevention in primary care

Under the scope of the primary care reform, patients will be cared for by interdisciplinary teams or by physician groups focusing on wellness and health promotion. The reform will comprise incentives to enhance comprehensive, coordinated care, particularly for chronic diseases, and focus on prevention.

The number of physicians participating in these models has increased remarkably: from 129 in February 2003 to approximately 2,000 in April 2004.

Sources and further reading:
First Ministers' Health Care Accord 2003: www.hc-sc.gc.ca/english/hca2003/accord.html
Ontario Family Health Network: www.ontariofamily healthnetwork.gov.on.ca/
Primary health care reform in selected other provinces: www.health.gov.sk.ca/ps_phs_services_over.html, www.healthservices.gov.bc.ca/phc/index.html

Public Health and Prevention

Total expenditures on prevention and public health as a percentage of GDP in network countries

	2001	2002
Australia	0.1	n/a
Austria	0.1	0.1
Canada	0.7	0.7
Denmark	n/a	n/a
Finland	0.2	0.3
France	0.2	0.2
Germany	0.5	0.5
Japan	0.2	n/a
Korea	0.1	n/a
Netherlands	0.4	0.4
New Zealand	n/a	n/a
Spain	0.1	0.1
Switzerland	0.3	0.2
United Kingdom	n/a	n/a
United States	0.6	0.6

OECD Health Data 2004

The following section describes examples of "classic" public health measures addressing major determinants of health as reported from California and South Korea.

It also presents three more comprehensive efforts: the Five-year Public Health Plan developped in France, the preparation of a public health law drawing on the recommendations of the second "Wanless Report" and subsequent consultations in England, and a law on health promotion launching the "Healthy Japan 21" campaign.

USA: Ban on soft drinks in schools

A recently published study indicated that obesity has overtaken smoking as the leading preventable cause of death in the United States. In California, 26 percent of school children are considered obese.

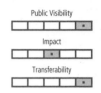

Public Visibility

Impact

Transferability

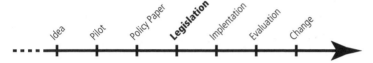

Idea · Pilot · Policy Paper · **Legislation** · Implementation · Evaluation · Change

In September 2003, the governor of California signed into law the California Childhood Obesity Prevention Act. Starting on July 1, 2004, this piece of legislation effectively locks soda and other high-sugar drinks out of public elementary, middle and junior high schools in California. It is the most comprehensive ban on unhealthy beverages in schools in the United States.

Obesity main preventable cause of death

Previous efforts to improve the nutritional environment for children in school always faltered because public schools depend heavily on fundraising activities to finance virtually everything from sports and after-school activities to school renovation. Nearly 60 percent of middle and high schools in the USA sell soft drinks via vending machines. A district may receive more than €800,000 per year with an exclusive contract. As the new law may cause serious financial shortfalls for many schools, it might become a major cause of contention. The public interest in both the health and the economic consequences thus remains high.

Schools in search of new funding sources

Sources and further reading:
Arizona State University—Commercialism in Education Research Unit: www.asu.edu/educ/epsl/CERU/CERU_2004_Research_Writing.htm

Medical Student JAMA: http://jama.ama-assn.org/cgi/content/full/288/17/2181

Associated Press. Californian Law Makers Ok Soda Ban for some Schools. August 22, 2003. www.cnn.com/2003/EDUCATION/08/22/sprj.sch.soda.ban.ap/.

Business Wire. California sends Soda Packing with Nations Most Comprehensive School Beverage Law. September 18, 2003. http://quickstart.clari.net/qs_se/webnews/wed/am/Bca-ccpha.Rhwv_DSI.html.

California Center for Public Health Advocacy. The California Childhood Obesity Prevention Act 2003. www.publichealthadvocacy.org/legislation/SB677_Summary.pdf.

California State Senate. SB677 - Senate Bill Analysis: info.sen.ca.gov/pub/bill/sen/sb_0651-0700/sb_677_cfa_20030822_112039_sen_floor.html.

Fried, Ellen J. und Marion Nestle. The Growing Political Movement Against Soft Drinks in Schools. Journal of the American Medical Association. (288) 2002: 2181. http://jama.ama-assn.org/cgi/content/full/288/17/2181.

South Korea: Tobacco tax increase proposal

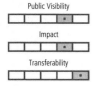

Public Visibility

Impact

Transferability

After attending the May 2003 WHO Health Assembly, where more active policies against smoking were strongly recommended, the Korean minister of health and welfare suggested raising the tobacco tax from €0.10 to €2.00.

The Ministry of Finance and Economy (MOFE) strongly opposed this plan, arguing that it would have a negative impact on tax revenue (of local governments) and exert inflationary pressure on the economy.

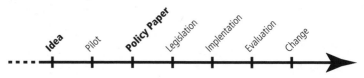

The decision on the level and timing of the tax increase was deliberately deferred until after general elections in April 2004. Facing strong opposition by the most powerful ministry (MOFE), the level of increase in tobacco tax will be smaller than originally proposed.

Sources and further reading:
Ministry of Health and Welfare: http://english.mohw.go.kr/index.jsp

England: Wanless Reports—health spending and public health

The first Wanless Report, commissioned by the Chancellor of the Exchequer, was published in April 2002. Sir Derek Wanless, former Group Chief Executive of National Westminster Bank, compiled this review of long-term funding needs of the NHS (National Health Service). The report showed that needs depend on the extent to which future funding demand for health care can be effectively reduced by sound public health policies.

In February 2004, a second report by Wanless, focusing on prevention and relevant health determinants in England, was published.

Public Visibility

Impact

Transferability

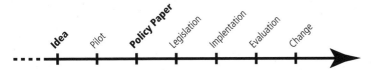

The second Wanless Report addresses common public health issues, such as smoking, obesity and health inequalities. Noting the need for more effective public health policies in these areas, the report attributes the lack of rigorous implementation not to a lack of information and knowledge but to the fact that acute care dominates the health care system. The report lists preconditions for more effective public health policies.

Acute care impairs application of effective prevention

The government has now announced a consultation period to gather proposals for discussion and debate that form the basis of an act. To ensure cost-effective use of resources, thorough monitoring and evaluation of public health measures is recommended.

Sources and further reading:
Wanless, Derek. Securing Good Health for the Whole Population. London: HM Treasury, 2004. www.hm-treasury.gov.uk/consultations_and_legislations/wanless/consult_wanless 03_index.cfm.
Wanless, Derek. Securing our Future Health: Taking a Long-term View. Final report. London: HM Treasury, 2002. www.hm-treasury.gov.uk/consultations_and_legislation/wanless/consult_wanless_ final.cfm.

France: Reform of the public health law

Public Visibility

Transferability

In May 2003, the government presented a bill to parliament to reform the French public health system and define public health measures and objectives for a five-year term (2004–2008). After a host of reviews and modifications, the bill was passed by the French assembly and presented to the senate in October 2003. After another series of amendments and a second reading, it was passed by the French assembly on August 9, 2004.

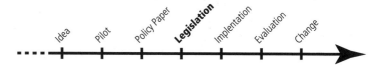

100 public health goals The law consists of five parts. The first two sections deal with definitions of national public health policy in France, institutions required to develop and implement this policy and ways to transfer the policy to the regional level. The third section describes 100 prioritized national public health goals grouped under umbrella issues, such as information policy, reduction of health inequalities and promotion of healthy nutrition, especially for children. Additionally, it outlines measures to achieve these goals and indicators to evaluate success.

40

Section four addresses research and professional training. The fifth section embraces a wider range of measures with regard to quality and performance of the entire public health system, the organization of professionals, etc.

What is remarkable about this reform is that at the beginning, most of the debates in the assembly as well as in the senate focused on public health objectives, although these objectives do not have any normative character. For most of them, indicators have not yet been defined. Preparation has only started, as national technical groups have been set up and are still working on this issue.

Seeking agreement on public health objectives

Sources and further reading:
Assemblée Nationale: Rapport au nom de la Commission des affaires culturelles, familiales et sociales sur le projet de loi, modifié par le Sénat, relatif à la politique de santé publique. www.assemblee-nationale.fr/12/rapports/r1473. asp.
Sénat. Project de Loi modifié par le Senat relatif à la politique de la santé publique. http://ameli.senat.fr/publica tion_pl/2003-2004/19.html.

Japan: Striving for "Healthy Japan 21"

In May 2003, the Japanese parliament passed a law on health promotion. The law provides a foundation for the philosophy and objectives of the health care strategy "Healthy Japan 21."

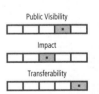

Public Visibility

Impact

Transferability

Japan's population is aging more rapidly than that of any other country in the world. This population shift entails major changes in the spectrum of diseases and consequently the needs in health care delivery (see also the chapter on aging in HPD 2/2003). These developments are expected to bring major increases in health care costs and a wider need for long-term care.

Drawing on the Healthy People 2000 campaign in the United States, Japan has now defined a series of health objectives.

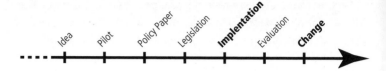

Idea   Pilot   Policy Paper   Legislation   **Implementation**   Evaluation   **Change**

One focal point of the law aims at standardizing the methods and documentation of preventive medical checkups. Up to now, these differed widely, and the records were not transferable (for example, if a person changed jobs). This made health information fragmented and difficult to compare. The health promotion law stipulates standardized procedures and documentation and provides every citizen with a booklet presenting the results, which also serves as a source of information.

The National Nutrition Survey, which is conducted every year to assess the actual intake of food, nutrients, etc. by nationals, is under revision aiming to prevent lifestyle-related diseases. In the meantime, nutritionists and managerial nutritionists are expected to manage not only meals, as they have done traditionally, but also people, as experts of nutrition.

Furthermore, the law requires all public spaces—such as schools, hospitals, public offices, restaurants, department stores, shops and public transportation—to be smoke-free. The managers of these facilities must take measures to protect people against passive smoking. The passage on prevention of passive smoking was the most controversial issue of this act. It raised strong opposition from smokers and the Japanese tobacco industry. However, as the law does not provide any penalties for failure to comply, implementation of this requirement is doubtful.

Sources and further reading:
Healthy Japan 21: www.nih.go.jp/eiken/english/research/ eiyo_top_e.html (in English), www.kenkounippon21.gr.jp/ index.html (in Japanese only)
Health Net: www.health-net.or.jp/index.html (in Japanese only)
Tobacco or Health: www.health-net.or.jp/tobacco/front. html (in Japanese only)

(Re-)Centralization versus Decentralization

In many countries, federal systems and subsidiary organizations for health services delivery and other social services are well established. More recently, Denmark, Finland, Spain and Switzerland report reforms aimed at modifying or amending the existing structures. There is a trend toward strengthening midlevel administration and/or reinforcing the normative and control functions of central health authorities or the ministry of health. **Safeguarding social standards**

Denmark is debating efficiency and quality concerns within the broader context of public administration and the future role of the counties. Also to enhance efficiency, in 2003 Finland launched a 10-year experiment in the Kainuu region to test a merger of educational, health, and other welfare services at a newly established county level to eventually replace competences traditionally located at the municipal level. A comparable trend can be observed in Switzerland, where the national government intervenes to adjust intercantonal inequalities by setting national targets.

In Spain, upon completion of a long journey toward regional autonomy and decentralization of health care competencies, the government today strives to ensure equal access and equity across Spanish regions, as decentralization has led to increased disparities.

Denmark: Strategy for the health care system—the patient

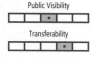
In December 2003, the Danish government presented a new strategy to maintain high-quality care in the health care sector. The strategy foresees measures to reduce waiting times and to provide patients with better information on hospitals. To achieve this, the government proposes to publish data on hospital performance ("yardstick competition"), to develop a set of indicators within a Danish Model for Quality and to honor high-quality achievements with financial rewards and with a performance-related increase in managerial autonomy.

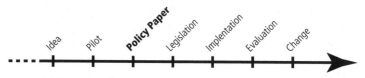

Administrative structures determine quality

The reform refers to an ongoing and still not finalized public administration reform that may change the number and size of counties. Depending on the scope and range of changes in administrative structure, the plans are likely to meet with fierce resistance from the counties.

The current minister of health initiated the idea in an attempt to introduce a Danish style of managed competition between counties as payers and between hospitals.

Finland: County-level management of welfare services

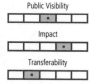
In June 2003, Finland launched a long-term administrative experiment in the northeastern region of Kainuu (one of the 20 regions that make up the six Finnish provinces). The size of Belgium, Kainuu region only has 85,000 inhabitants. The population is aging and diminishing, and unemployment is high. Municipalities will probably not be able to provide the full range of social and welfare services to their residents in the future.

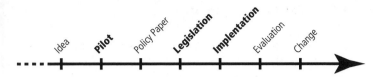

Idea · Pilot · Policy Paper · Legislation · Implementation · Evaluation · Change

Centralization— solution for sparsely populated areas?

Designed to run over a period of ten years, the experiment sets out to create a new self-regulating administrative level above the municipal level. It is expected to be functional as of January 1, 2005.

The new entity will receive and manage all financial and human resources that were previously channeled to the municipal authorities. Most of the municipalities of the Kainuu region agreed to participate in this experiment. But as independence of municipalities has a long tradition in Finland, the move toward greater centralization will markedly change the administration and provision of welfare services. Some municipalities were reluctant to participate because they would lose control over administrative processes and the allocation of funds. However, integration of services met little opposition. On the whole, debate was scant, with little media coverage.

The pooling of competencies, funds and manpower on an upper administrative level is expected to contribute to the integration of social and health care services and to strengthen economic development and cooperation in the Kainuu region. The impact of the new self-administration will be tested and evaluated as a potentially sustainable solution for the future.

Sources and further reading:
Leskinnen, Hannu. The Regional Self-Government Experiment in the Kainuu Region. www.kainuu.fi/kainuunliitto/ Hallintokokeilu/Yleista/Self-government%20experiment %20in%20Kainuu.pdf.

Austria: Health purchasing agencies

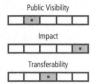

In May 2004, the Austrian Ministry of Health announced the creation of health purchasing agencies (HPAs): regionally operating organizations to consolidate financing and accountability in the provision of inpatient care and ambulatory care.

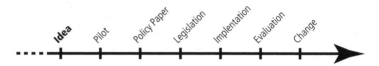

Financing and accountability of health service provision in Austria is currently split across stakeholders. As a result of vertical and horizontal fragmentation of service provision, remuneration is funded by separate sources. Reflecting a single-payer approach, HPAs are expected to optimize resource allocation by improving coordination and cooperation and to facilitate a purchaser-provider split in the hospital sector.

HPAs—a constitutional shift

To enhance the integration of service delivery, the agencies will be composed of representatives from social security, local governments and the federal government. If approved, this policy would generate and require subsequent constitutional amendments, as the allocation of the balance of power between payers is concerned. As it stands, HPAs would have considerable impact on the Austrian health care system. Developed with very little involvement of important stakeholders, it will likely meet fierce resistance.

Sources and further reading:
Government program: http://www2.oeaab.at/wien/archiv/INHALT/regierung.html (Regierungsprogramm der Österreichischen Bundesregierung für die XXII. Gesetzgebungsperiode)
Bundesministerium für Gesundheit und Frauen. Die österreichische Gesundheitsreform 2005, Themenfeld Verbesserung der Effizienz und nachhaltige Sicherung der Finanzierung im Gesundheitswesen. May 2004.

Switzerland: Improving territorial equity in a federal state

In December 2003, the Swiss parliament rejected the second revision of the Health Insurance Act (HPD 2/2003). In March 2004, the Federal Council (Swiss government) decided not to modify the content of the reform but to choose a different, rather unconventional approach to achieve its goals. The reform proposal is now divided into two bills containing six small packages, which can be passed by parliament in an accelerated process (see also Newsflash in this issue, p. 63 ff.). The first bill contains a package that aims at improving territorial equity. The Federal Council submitted the first reform proposal in March 2004 for debate during the autumnal session of the Swiss parliament starting in September 2004.

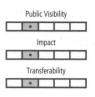

Public Visibility

Impact

Transferability

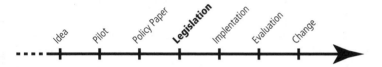

In Switzerland, compulsory health insurance is financed by per-capita premiums. To partly compensate for the resulting inequity of financing, state subsidies for low-income persons were introduced in 1996 under the Health Insurance Act. Two thirds of these subsidies are borne by the federal authorities of the Swiss confederation (the Confederation), one third by the cantons.

26 different canton subsidy schemes

Because the cantons autonomously determine the specific regulations for premium subsidies, this system features 26 different arrangements and pronounced inequalities.

Various approaches exist to calculate the income of the insured (gross, net and taxable respectively). Eligibility for premium subsidies is differentiated by income categories or triggered when the amount paid for premiums exceeds a certain percentage of income. Some cantons give financial support automatically, while others provide the subsidy only if the insured person applies for it. Some cantons pass the subsidy on to the health insurers; others pay it directly to the insured. The premiums for children also vary from canton to canton. Subsidies differ in levels as well as in number of children supported.

To improve equity across the country as well as vertical equity within the population, the Swiss national government introduced the following measures:

The economic situation of people eligible for subsidies shall be defined accurately and in a uniform way. To assess the insured person's economic situation (i.e., ability to pay), nationwide standards shall be introduced. For each canton a reference premium would be defined and a maximum share of income (specifically, family income) to be spent on health insurance premiums specified. In the lowest income class—which could still be defined by the cantons—, premiums would not exceed four percent of income for singles or couples and two percent for families with children; for the highest income group, the figures are 10 and 12 percent respectively. Eligibility for subsidies and assessment of economic situation are still under discussion.

The Confederation promised to provide an additional €127 million to implement the reform, which the cantons consider to be too little. Beyond that, the cantons oppose the reform for three major reasons: The proposal represents a certain centralization of devolved health policy competencies from the cantons to the central government; the Confederation does not adjust the annual federal subsidies to cost changes; and the distribution of federal subsidies should take into account not only the canton's population and financial strength, but also the average cantonal premium.

Sources and further reading:
Eidgenössisches Departement des Innern. Krankenversicherung: Bundesrat stellt Reformplanung vor. Press release. February 25, 2004. www.edi.admin.ch/presse/2004/040225_kvg-reformplanung.pdf.
Eidgenössisches Departement des Innern. Krankenversicherung: Bundesrat verabschiedet
Vernehmlassungsvorlage. Press release. March 24, 2004. www.edi.admin.ch/presse/2004/040324_kvg-vernehmlassung.pdf.

Spain: Evaluating regional health care financing

In 2002, health care management competence was transferred to ten regional governments (HPD 1/2003). The other seven regions had already gained autonomy in this area during the 1990s. At the same time, responsibilities for financing health services were passed to the regions as well.

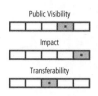

Public Visibility

Impact

Transferability

To finance health care, the regional governments draw on three types of resources: their own taxes, shared taxes and transfers from the central government. In addition, extra assignments aim to compensate for regional disparities arising from unexpected demographic changes. Two years after adoption, this chapter provides an interim evaluation.

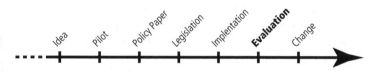

Idea   Pilot   Policy Paper   Legislation   Implementation   **Evaluation**   Change

Since fiscal co-accountability was introduced in 2002, health care expenditures have increased for three consecutive years. Even though the trend seems to be slowing, all regional budgets for health care have increased at a higher rate than the GDP.

Striking increase in health care expenditure

The average per-capita budget rose from €923 in 2003 to €955 in 2004, that is, by approximately 3.5 percent. Differences between the regions are quite remarkable, at up to €440 per capita (La Rioja €1227 and Baleares €787 per capita).

Pharmaceutical invoices and higher personnel costs are the main factors behind this trend. The definition of a common minimum benefit basket under the National Cohesion Act has also contributed, as have other efforts, to ensure equal access to health care. In addition, the reform may have produced more inefficiency because of increased transaction costs for cooperation and coordination of services.

Interfering reasons are hampering the assessment

Sources and further reading:

Cantarero, David: Análisis del gasto sanitario autonómico y su nueva financiación en España. Investigaciones, nffl 7/03, Instituto de Estudios Fiscales, Madrid, 2003.

Cantarero, David, and Rosa Urbanos: Políticas sectoriales de gasto público: Sanidad. In Salinas, Javier, and Santiago Álvarez (eds.): El gasto público en la democracia. Estudios en el XXV aniversario de la Constitución Española de 1978. Instituto de Estudios Fiscales, Madrid, 2003.

López i Casasnovas, Guillem: La capitación en la financiación territorial de los servicios públicos transferidos: El caso de la sanidad y de la educación. Mffl Sanidad, Madrid, 1999.

Tamayo, Pedro Antonio: Descentralización y financiación de la asistencia sanitaria pública en España. Un estudio desde la perspectiva de la equidad. Colección Estudios CES, Madrid, 2001.

Urbanos, Rosa, and Alfonso Utrilla: La financiación de los servicios sanitarios: Distribución de fondos por CCAA y efectos sobre la suficiencia dinámica. In Salinas, Javier (ed.): El nuevo modelo de financiación autonómica, pp. 161-202, Estudios de Hacienda Pública, Instituto de Estudios Fiscales, Madrid, 2002.

New Zealand: Interim evaluation of District Health Boards

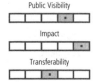

In 2001, the public health system in New Zealand was restructured and 21 District Health Boards (DHBs) were established. They are currently under review. The DHBs are funded on a per-capita district-level base. Based on a needs assessment, DHBs purchase or provide health services to their population. All DHB decisions, action and strategic plans must be in line with the national health strategy.

DHBs were introduced to anchor a population-based focus in the public health system in order to make the system more responsive, to improve district-level cooperation, and to increase community participation in decision making.

DHBs are somewhat similar to the organizations responsible for the health care system in New Zealand prior to 1993. After major reforms during the nineties aiming at an increased market orientation, in 1999 the newly elected labor-led government restructured the system again by introducing DHBs.

An interim report of the evaluation team describes some key findings. DHBs enjoy broad general support, but many experts think there are too many of them, leading to a fragmentation of the critical mass of expertise. Board elections may produce imbalances in skill mix or ethnic constitution that must be compensated for. The holding of elections every three years is likely to advance instability. Performance monitoring through the government is regarded as intrusive and costly.

Costly micro-management

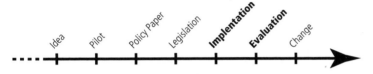

The Ministry has sometimes shown some reluctance to devolve decision-making and funding competencies to the 21 districts. Non-government providers are concerned about accountability mechanisms, problems and costs of having to work with several DHBs. Nevertheless, the debate is rather consensual.

The most relevant driver of DHBs was the politicians' belief that the community ought to participate in health sector decision making. However, community involvement is not associated with greater equity in the health care system.

Persuasion rather than evidence

Sources and further reading:
Devlin, Nancy, Alan Maynard, and Nicholas Mays: New Zealand's new health sector reforms: back to the future? *British Medical Journal* (322) 2001: 1171-1174.
Health Reforms 2001 Research Team. Interim Report 2001 on Health Reforms 2001 Research Project. www.vuw.ac.nz/hsrc/reports/downloads/Interim%20Report%20on%20Health%20Reforms%202001.pdf

Technical Innovations and Bioethics

Reports from Denmark and Spain address the use of information technologies (IT) in each health care system. Comprehensive IT solutions are regarded as a tool to improve cooperation and coordination across the health care system and at the interface to the social care system, thus offering a possibility to mobilize cost-efficiency reserves.

Surveys from France and Singapore report on the highly contentious issue of bioethics. When it comes to the ethical and moral fundament on which the debate is based, it is often regarded as too complicated to be discussed and judged in public.

To adopt European Union legislation and with pressure to update a law from 1994, France is debating a revision of the legislative framework on bioethics. Issues such as organ transplants, medically assisted reproduction, therapeutic cloning, and genes patenting are all on the lawmakers' agenda. During a lengthy process, the originally research-oriented approach of the previous center-left government gave way to a rather conservative one under the center-right government. As the French regional elections held in March 2004 brought an explicit change in powers, the approach may shift again.

Singapore amended its transplantation act to overcome the shortage in organ donations.

Denmark: Electronic patient records in hospitals

In 2003, the Danish government issued a document called "National IT strategy for the health care sector 2003-2007." The paper describes several initiatives aimed at improving the coordination of information technologies (IT), promoting state-of-the-art use of IT throughout Denmark by applying national standards, and introducing electronic patient records (EPR) in all hospitals by the end of 2005.

EPRs facilitate the exchange of information not only among health care providers but also between providers and patients. A Web site established in December 2003 collects information about health status and health care and serves as a platform for the exchange of (confidential) patient information. The vision is that patients will have access to their own records, too.

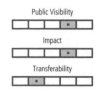

IT to cover health sector by 2005

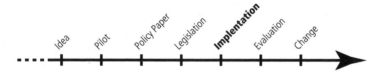

As general practitioners have already been using EPRs for the past ten years, compatibility among their different systems is a major challenge still unsolved.

To encourage the introduction of EPRs in the hospital sector, financial incentives (e.g., a lump-sum grant) were built into the budget agreement between counties and the central government. Criticism arises mainly because of the timeframe, which hospitals that are just beginning to use IT regard as too narrow. Further concerns affect the increased powers of central administration.

Sources and further reading:
Danish health system: www.sundhed.dk (in Danish only)

Spain: Electronic drug management

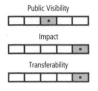

Public Visibility

Impact

Transferability

IT to improve quality of drug prescription

In 2003, the Cohesion and Quality of the National Health System Act (HPD 1/2003) set the frame for electronic prescribing, dispensing and invoicing. In 2004, feasibility of electronic drug management is explicitly included in the Act Accompanying the Budget of the Central Government for 2004, thus amending the Law of Drugs.

Electronic drug management serves a range of purposes. It is introduced to increase the information on drug prescription through a central data bank, to link all providers involved in the management of drugs, and to improve the quality of patient information on any given drug. It is also expected to reduce bureaucracy and to increase control over prescriptions and expenditure.

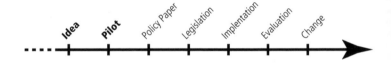

Since 2000, several pilot projects on electronic prescriptions (e.g., PISTA I/II, Gaia, Receta XXI) have been implemented. Most of them work on a regional level (GAIA in Valencia, RECETA XXI in Andalusia), but some have already started to connect different regions (PISTA: Madrid, Catalonia, Canary Islands, Basque Provinces). Experience from the pilot projects will feed into nationwide legislation on electronic prescriptions.

Ethical concerns

A number of ethical concerns remain to be solved: privacy issues for patients and providers, limited freedom of physicians and pharmacists and misuse as an instrument for cost containment.

Sources and further reading:
Ministerio de Sanidad y Consumo: www.msc.es
Cohesion and Quality of the National Health System Act: www.agemed.es/legislacion/espana/pdf/RCL_2003_1412 Vigente.pdf (in Spanish only)

France: Bioethics legislation

In France, a new legislative framework, adopted August 6, 2004, re-regulates issues such as organ donation, medically assisted reproduction, therapeutic cloning and gene patenting. The new law enacts ethical principles, defines what is meant by "crime against the human species" as a new category of crimes. It provides a list of forbidden research activities (e.g., research on or production of stem cells) and permitted research activities (e.g., transitory projects on cells made available by medically assisted procreation), a list of control bodies overseeing the biosciences, and foresees severe penal sanctions for breaking the new laws.

Public Visibility

Impact

Transferability

Overall, the planned framework is based on sanctions rather than incentives. Following the traditional French approach, the content of the legislation relies on reports and advice from "qualified individuals" and their personal value sets. Policy makers did not encourage a wider public debate or use evidence to shape the bill.

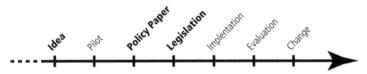

The legislation on reproduction and transplantation is not controversial. Regulation of medically assisted reproduction is straightforward, and the new regulation on organ donations is expected to increase the number of available organs. Once technical requirements are met, individuals must explicitly state their disagreement to avoid organ withdrawal after their death. This provision sharply contrasts with, for instance, the German human organ transplant act, where family members and spouses have a say if the deceased had not explicitly approved the donation of organs.

Whose body is it?

55

Brain drain in biotech research?

A major issue is the ban on therapeutic cloning. Between January 2002 and January 2003, the draft was dramatically altered in the parliamentary process from a rather open attitude toward new biotechnologies and their use to a coercive and limitative one. Opponents fear that this approach will considerably impede biological research in France, resulting in a brain drain and fewer patents on biological inventions.

Another delicate topic is gene patenting. France was required to implement EU directive 98/44/EC. The French government chose to comply with the directive in order to open and facilitate political renegotiation. Conservative opponents fear that negotiations will not be resumed and that the human genome may be sold out to the private market.

Can ethical norms be evaluated?

Evaluation has been dismissed as inappropriate. According to the official government argument, issues as supreme as ethical values must not be submitted to "real world" criteria. All the same, negotiation of this issue behind closed doors may merely increase uncertainty, generate defensiveness, and thereby impede a sustainable societal solution. However, an evaluation of the stem cell research projects authorized for a transitory period of five years will be conducted at the end of this period.

Sources and further reading:
Comité Consultatif National d'Ethique pour les sciences de la vie et de la santé: www.ccne-ethique.fr/francais/start.htm (in French only)
Parliamentary debates in the National Assembly: www.assemblee-nat.fr/12/cri/2003-2004/ (in French only)
Projet de loi relatif à la bioéthique: www.senat.fr/doslegman/pjl01-189_travaux.html (in French only)
Gros, François. Les cellules souches adultes et leurs potentialites d'utilisation en recherche et en therapeutique. Comparaison avec les cellules souches embryonnaires. Rapport établi à la demande de Roger-Gérard Schwartzenberg, ministre de la Recherche. www.ladocumentation francaise.fr/brp/notices/014000287.shtml.
Lalande, Françoise, Valérie Delahaye-Guillocheau, Marc Ollivier and Elisabeth Dufourcq. Conservation d'éléments

du corps humain en milieu hospitalier. http://lesrapports. ladocumentationfrancaise.fr/BRP/024000374/0000.pdf. Office parlementaire d'èvaluation des choix scientifiques et technologiques. Rapport sur l'application de la loi n 94-654 du 29 juillet 1994 relative au don et à l'utilisation des éléments et produits du corps humain, à l'assistance médicale à la procréation et au diagnostic prénatal. www.assemblee-nat.fr/rap-oecst/bioethique/r1407-01. asp#_Toc443973735.

Singapore: Amendments to the Human Organ Transplant Act

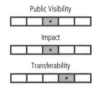

Public Visibility

Impact

Transferability

In January 2004, the Singaporean parliament passed amendments to the Human Organ Transplant Act after a broad public consultation exercise (HPD 1/2003).

Two pieces of legislation deal with human organ transplantation. The Medical Therapy Education and Research Act sets forth an opt-in system. People can pledge their organs for transplantation, medical education or research after they die. Relatives may also donate organs of brain-dead patients who did not make this pledge.

Opting in or opting out?

The other law, the Human Organ Transplant Act, describes an opt-out system. Previously, the law provided only for the kidneys of traffic accident victims to be used for transplantation, except if the person had opted out of the system. The amendments recently passed extended the range of the law greatly. The permission to transplant organs is now extended to liver, heart and cornea; organs may be taken after all causes of death; and both cadaver organ donation and organ donation by living donors are allowed.

The organ transplant waitlist

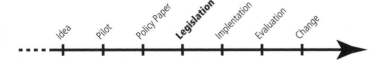

There was no noteworthy controversy during the legislative process. The issue of whether to choose an opt-in or opt-out system was the main topic of discussion. The opt-out system was maintained, and the Ministry of Health will inform affected persons about their rights.

Sources and further reading:
Ministry of Health Singapore: www.moh.gov.sg/corp/systems/organ/hota/faqs.do
Medical Protection Society Singapore. New rules for organ transplants: www.medicalprotection.org/Medical/Singapore/News/News/20040130_hota.aspx.

Newsflash

In the United States, insurance coverage gaps continue to expand. The economic downturn and other factors have put pressure on the funding of health care for the entire population.

Besides recurrent discussions on uniform and universal coverage (HPD 1/2003), measures to ration and reduce health care are also high on the agenda (in California and Oregon). The aims of these reforms are contradictory. On the one hand, states seek to curb the high costs of emergency services by expanding entitlement to state-funded medical plans. On the other hand, different measures aim to keep the number of eligible persons low. California legislators are even risking a quarrel with the mighty pharmaceutical industry to contain drug cost expenditures.

Another intriguing topic is the creative way the Swiss government has dealt with the Health Insurance Act rejected in a 2003 referendum. To avoid further delays, the Swiss government divided the rejected reform package into separate bills, to be passed by parliament by way of an accelerated process in which no further referenda are needed. Otherwise, another referendum might have called for a start from scratch. Meanwhile, some legislative decrees would have expired. The obligation to draft a new bill would have delayed any reform process for many years.

The World Health Report 2000 ranked France in the first place of 191 health care systems with respect to overall system performance. Since then, the picture might well have changed: Two high-profile reports—the Chadelat Report (HPD 2/2003) and in response the report of the Haut Conseil pour l'avenir de l'assurance maladie (High Council on the future of sickness insurance)—indicate that France is discussing fundamental changes in health care funding.

USA: Oregon Health Plan cuts

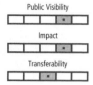

Public Visibility

Impact

Transferability

In April 2004, the Oregon Department of Human Services (DHS) presented a budget plan to abolish state health insurance coverage for the "working poor"—people who do not qualify for Medicaid. Medicaid is a partnership matching funds program between federal and state governments to ensure a minimum level of health coverage for the most vulnerable populations.

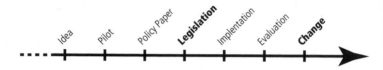

The Oregon scheme, much valued, ...

Originally, the Oregon Health Plan (OHP) sought to provide uniform, universal coverage to both those eligible for Medicaid and the working poor. To achieve this, planners developed a prioritized list of health services defined by a broad spectrum of stakeholders. Based on a range of prioritized conditions coupled with their most effective treatments, the list was used to ration health services according to the previously determined agreements with providers.

... went bankrupt

At the outset, the plan worked well. However, rising costs and the sluggish economy between 2001 and 2003 triggered a series of cost-cutting measures and reforms (OHP 2). Adding to the fact that health care costs were rising, many managed-care plans pulled out of the OHP, forcing the state to buy fee-for-service arrangements that further increased costs. During FY 2003/ 2004, the budget crisis worsened again, and the government's attempt to preserve the coverage and the spirit of the OHP failed. As voters, federal regulators or health care providers blocked additional funding, the DHS created a budget-cutting plan. This plan will completely eliminate the working poor from coverage and use the "savings" to buy back some services that were on the state's priority list but not federally mandated.

While it is still unclear to what extent the DHS plan will be realized, the proposal is perceived as a signal announcing the end of the Oregon experiment to provide health insurance coverage to a broader share of the population.

Sources and further reading:
The Henry J. Kaiser Family Foundation, Commission on Medicaid and the Uninsured: www.kff.org/about/kcmu.cfm
Oregon Health Plan: www.dhs.state.or.us/healthplan/

California: Update on employer mandate for health insurance

An alliance of business groups is actively pursuing legislative and legal attacks to block implementation of the Health Insurance Act of 2003. Opponents initiated a referendum, Californians against Government-Run Health Care, which will appear on the November 2004 ballot.

Public Visibility

Impact

Transferability

In his last few days of office, Governor Grey Davis signed SB-2 into law (HPD 2/2003). The Health Insurance Act of 2003 stipulates that employers must provide health coverage or pay a fee to the state, which would then obtain the coverage. Terms vary according to business size, with considerably less required of smaller businesses. A coalition of unions, health advocates and insurers supported the law, which extended coverage to approximately one million uninsured Californians.

Extending coverage to one million uninsured

As the annual cost of insurance reaches approximately €3,321 for an individual and more than €7,472 for a family, opponents argue this may endanger economic and job growth as well as existing insurance coverage, which is likely to be scaled back.

Soaring health costs slow down growth

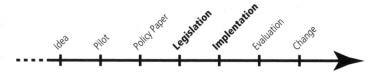

The employer insurance mandate limits dependence on state revenues. A commission was established to address cost-containment measures, and subsidies for smaller businesses are recommended. However, none of these measures is state-funded.

Employer
mandate
hard-fought
On the national as well as on the state level, there have been many attempts to implement universal coverage. However, this has always been a very contentious issue and vulnerable to political and economic changes.

In California, in particular, the debate is very controversial; it remains to be seen whether the Health Insurance Act of 2003 will stand.

> *Sources and further reading:*
> Griffin, Sarah Heck, and Brian T. Holmen. Jones Day Commentaries. California Senate Bill 2 (2003). www1.jonesday.com/pubs/detail.asp?language=English&pubid=1153, March 2004.

California: Prescription drug reimportation legislation

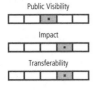

Public Visibility

Impact

Transferability

In April 2004, both houses of the California legislature passed reimportation legislation. The bill aims to lower the costs for prescription drugs by enabling private consumers and state agencies to purchase US-manufactured drugs from Canada. The strategy, called reimportation, is highly controversial. Opponents cite concerns about patient safety and the threat to biomedical innovation.

Addressing the major factor boosting health care costs

Between 1996 and 2003, state expenditures on prescription drugs rose by about 350 percent. Prescription drug costs represent an expanding share of declining health care budgets.

Purchasers who take advantage of Canadian price controls and the beneficial exchange rate can reduce drug costs by 30 to 60 percent. To facilitate private purchasing while protecting consumers, a state-run Web site will list Canadian pharmacies certified as safe by the California board of pharmacies.

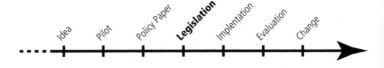

Federal law prohibits the reimportation of drugs. However, seven states have some kind of scheme to bypass the regulations. So far, none of these measures has been penalized. The pharmaceutical industry is exerting enormous pressure, spending huge sums of money and positioning more than 600 lobbyists in Washington to influence national policy.

A billion dollars spent to keep drug prices up

Members of the California senate and assembly who introduced the bill are committed to low-cost health care and affordable prescription drugs for all Californians. This highly contentious issue has divided various interest groups, such as physician organizations. The California Medical Association (CMA) supports the bill, while the American Medical Association (AMA) opposes it.

The outcome of the process remains doubtful, as the industry has taken very strong measures. Large pharmaceutical companies have already reduced shipments to foreign countries or announced that they will restrict sales to quantities sufficient for domestic use in each country.

Showing teeth

Sources and further reading:
The Henry J. Kaiser Family Foundation: www.kff.org
The California Health Care Foundation: www.chcf.org
The California Health Care Institute: www.chi.org

Switzerland: Individual passage of the reforms of the health insurance act

The Swiss parliament rejected the second revision of the health insurance law in December 2003 (HPD 2/2003), with the decision-making process rather than the law's contents as the leading cause of failure. Consequently, in February 2004 the Federal Council of Switzerland (Swiss government) decided to take another approach to implementing the various proposals.

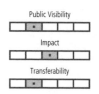

Public Visibility

Impact

Transferability

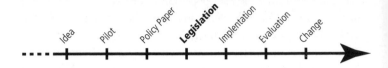

The reform act addressed a large number of heterogeneous topics. The wide range of issues made it nearly impossible to achieve agreement on the revision as a whole. In addition, the fact that at least one of the reform topics (selective contracting) was strongly opposed publicly made it very likely that a popular ballot would have been initiated. Such a referendum would have set back any endeavor to reform the health insurance act by years.

Old wine in new bottles   The reform now comes as a set of more manageable packages, each of which can be assessed separately and passed by parliament in an accelerated procedure.

The main topics of the health insurance act are subdivided into three acts. The first addresses the following issues in particular: maximum incidence levels for health insurance, free contracting, increased co-payments, and less regulated deductibles. Discussion began in March 2004; the bill will go to parliament in summer 2004 and probably become law between January and July 2005. The second proposal concerns encouragement of managed-care models and the provisional reorganization of hospital financing. Debate on this proposal will commence in the fall of 2004. Finally, the reorganization of financing for long-term care will be discussed starting in December 2004.

Sources and further reading:
Eidgenössisches Departement des Innern. Krankenversicherung: Bundesrat stellt Reformplanung vor. Press release. February 25, 2004. www.edi.admin.ch/presse/ 2004/040225_kvg-reformplanung.pdf.
Eidgenössisches Departement des Innern. Krankenversicherung: Bundesrat verabschiedet Vernehmlassungsvorlage. Press release. March 24, 2004. www.edi.admin.ch/presse/2004/040324_kvg-vernehmlassung.pdf.

According to present law, all medical professionals authorized to practice their independent profession in Switzerland automatically have access to a frame contract with all sickness funds. In the future, most European medical practitioners will fall into this category.

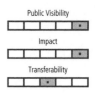

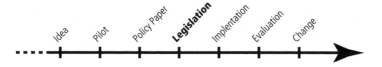

Providers are reimbursed through a fee-for-service scheme. The organizational context makes the Swiss health care system the most expensive in Europe and threatens its sustainability. During the discussion of the revision of the health insurance law, an abolition of compulsory contracting was proposed and finally rejected. However, a moratorium limiting the number of new physicians was decreed in July 2002. This moratorium expires in mid-2005.

Freedom of contract

The freedom of contract under the new law does not refer merely to the choice of partners. It has also to do with the contract's contents; the duration of the contract, the conditions for giving notice and even the fees will be subject to individual negotiation.

Quality of care and equity of access endangered

While the cantons would retain the responsibility for ensuring supply, the Federal Council will fix the minimum and maximum numbers of providers. As mentioned above, this issue was the most contentious, triggering fierce debate by physicians' associations, the insurance association Santésuisse and the public.

Sources and further reading:
Health Insurance Act: www.admin.ch/ch/d/sr/832_103/index.html (in German, French and Italian)
Crivelli, Luca, Massimo Filippini and Ilaria Mosca. Federalismo e spesa sanitaria regionale: analisi empirica per i Cantoni svizzeri. www.bul.unisi.ch/cerca/bul/pubblicazioni/eco/pdf/wp0304.pdf.

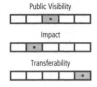

Public Visibility

Impact

Transferability

Every person living in Switzerland is subject to mandatory health insurance. Premiums are capitation-based; the levels depend on the place of residence and the insurance company. In addition, the insured participate in the costs of treatment in two ways. First, they pay an annual deductible, at present fixed at €200. After this, they pay a co-payment: 10 percent of the entailed expenses exceeding the deductible, up to a maximum of €450 per year. The insured may reduce the insurance premiums by choosing higher deductibles. The terms of these options are highly regulated.

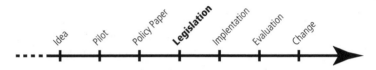

Increasing co-payments

The Swiss government plans to double co-payments from 10 to 20 percent while retaining the ceiling at €450. Furthermore, a liberalization of the optional-deductible system is envisioned.

In spite of the significant private contribution of the population to health care expenses (approx. 30 percent of health care expenses), moral hazard is suspected. Higher deductibles and increased co-payments are supposed to scale back infelicitous use of health care services.

Sources and further reading:
Bundesamt für Gesundheit. Statistik der obligatorischen Krankenversicherung 2002. Bern 2004. www.bag.admin. ch/kv/statistik/d/2004/KV_2002.pdf.
Bundesamt für Sozialversicherung. Die Franchisen 1997–2001. Eine Längsschnittanalyse über die Entwicklung der wählbaren Jahresfranchisen. Bern 2003. www.bag.admin. ch/kv/statistik/d/Franchisen97_01_D.pdf.

France: High Council on the future of sickness insurance

The French government that took office in 2002 announced a constitutional health care reform process, to start in the fall of 2003.

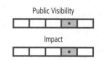
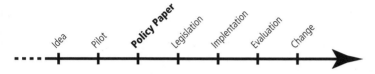

The Haut Conseil pour l'avenir de l'assurance maladie (High Council on the future of sickness insurance) was asked to diagnose the current health care system, consult and debate with all relevant stakeholders and present a draft reform to be discussed in summer 2004. The council was modeled after the very effective Pension Stewardship Council that prepared the French pension schemes reform.

Stakeholder consultation process

Members of the High Council represent all relevant interest groups, namely parliament, workers unions, employers unions, the state, sickness funds, supplementary insurers, health professionals in private practice, public and private hospitals, patients associations and renowned specialists.

Taking the lead in public debate on the reform process, the High Council is expected to raise the quality of debate, thus leading to enhanced acceptance of health care reform. It remains to be seen whether stakeholders really give up their own interests in order to attain a corporate, sustainable solution. The election result of the French regional elections in March 2004 was regarded as a slap in the face to the national French government.

Will the High Council achieve its aims?

Sources and further reading:
Ministry of Health: www.sante.gouv.fr

International Monitor on Health Policy Developments[1] Questionnaire

The approach

Overall goals

Does health policy reform work? How and why? This is what this questionnaire intends to explore. The focus of this survey is therefore on
- the analysis of the common features of health policy and health care reform across industrialized countries; and on
- the sequential analysis of health policy ideas, change processes and change management in health policy. Particular attention will be paid to key players, their interactions and on stewardship in health policy as a factor of change.

Network objectives

- To obtain and analyze information on changes and developments in health sector reform on a regular basis and over time
- To scout, monitor and follow a (new) health policy idea or approach from its inception stage through the policy and law-making process to implementation
- To describe and analyze the formal and informal interactions of all players and stakeholders at each stage in the decision-making process
- To capture best practice models already established

---

1 The term "Health Policy Development" has been chosen to capture both active reform processes (e.g., laws and acts) as well as technological and/or organizational changes with their implications for health policy. Similarly, the term "development" encompasses the various stages of a "health policy idea" from its inception or appearance via acceptance, adoption and implementation to decay, abandonment or change.

What we want to do with it

- To establish an effective tool for monitoring innovative ideas as they evolve and travel within and across health care systems
- To systematically analyze decision-making processes leading to health sector reforms or facilitating change in health policy
- To review and disseminate that information in an efficient, straightforward and rapid manner among all network partners (half-yearly reports, Internet platform)
- To organize the transfer of findings and results into the German health policy making process (consultations, advisory activities)

A word of caution

We do not seek to provide health system descriptions for the countries participating in this network. For most network countries, comprehensive health system descriptions do already exist. We particularly recognize the country studies developed and published by the European Observatory on Health Care Systems, the "Health Care Systems in Transition" (HiT) profiles. HiTs exist for 12 out of currently 16 network countries (for Canada, the report is from 1996 though). For Japan and the OECD, OECD Labour Market and Social Policy Occasional Papers are similarly comprehensive. For Singapore and South Korea, other suitable documents have been identified.

Structure of this survey

In each survey phase covering six months, we will ask you to provide information on the progress of a health policy idea, approach or instrument from the early stage of inception towards implementation over time.

For every six-month period, you will be asked to describe five or more such key health policy developments, selected according to the four criteria mentioned below. We are interested in comparing the background/context of a key health policy issue, its players/process interactions, and, with a view to implementation, its potential impact. The criteria for selection of a health policy development are:

- Relevance and scope
- Impact on status quo
- Degree of innovation (compared with national and international standards)
- Media coverage/Public attention

We are particularly interested in those reforms with significant impact on the overall structure and organization of your country's health system.

The questionnaire (one each for each of the selected health policy developments) starts with a two-dimensional matrix, picturing key issues (14 categories) and their development over time (seven process stages). For each of the selected key health policy issues, we will ask you to provide a more detailed analysis of stakeholders and their interests and interactions along the stages of the process. The matrix will allow you to categorize both the issue addressed and the current stage of the process.

It is possible that some ideas evolve very fast from one stage to the next. You may also observe that others do not necessarily follow the process, "surfacing" in at stage 2 and/or "jumping" across various stages during the period observed.

Matrix—First dimension: Issue clusters[2]

1. Sustainable financing of health care systems:
This cluster has been divided into "funding and pooling of funds" and "remuneration and paying providers," i.e., the relationship between population/patients and payers on the one side and between payers/purchasers and providers on the other. The first sub-section includes generation and collection of funds for health care (i.e., taxes, social insurance contributions or copayments) as well as their pooling and (re-)distribution to the payers (sickness funds or health authorities, including risk structure compensation). Important considerations relate to efficiency and equity. The second sub-section includes budgeting, diagnostic-related group (DRG) systems, drug pricing policy, etc.

2. Human resources:
Education and training, numbers and planning, projected shortages of qualified medical and non-medical personnel, etc.

3. Quality issues:
This should include tools such as guidelines, evidence-based medicine, peer reviews, re-certification of physicians, outcome measurements as well as measures to make them work (e. g., purchaser-provider contracts, financial/non-financial incentives), patient safety and medical errors/malpractice, public disclosure of provider performance data, benchmarks, best-practice.

---

2 The issue clusters in this matrix are a result of the kick-off meeting of the network participants in Germany in September 2002. In a brain-storming exercise, participants were asked to identify the current five major health policy challenges in their countries. The brain-storming was followed by a factor analysis grouping all issues raised in clusters/categories. The categories were completed during discussions and reorganized for survey purposes.

4. Benefit basket and priority setting:
This cluster includes both the decision-making process on (new) technologies and services, e.g., the question of whether health technology assessment becomes mandatory, as well as actual changes in the benefits covered, e.g., the exclusion of dental care.

5. Access:
In contrast to the previous cluster which deals with technologies and services, this cluster is about de facto access by individuals to health care, including problems such as rationing, waiting lists (equity concerns!), strategies for solving these restrictions and for reducing disparities in care.

6. Responsiveness and empowerment:
Responsiveness of the health care system and of health policy to patients, payers'[3] expectations, patient rights and patient charters.

7. Political context and public administration:
Refers to levels of competency (including EU), centralized vs. decentralized responsibilities, policy making styles, stewardship role, etc.[4]

8. Organization/integration of care across sectors:
This cluster incorporates developments that aim at the reconfiguration of health care providers, especially to overcome institutional and sectoral boundaries in order to provide disease management and other forms of integrated care.

9. Long-term care:
Long-term care and care for the elderly (aiming particularly at this group even if it also fits into one of the dimensions above).

10. Role of private sector:
This cluster deals with developments that specifically aim at changing (regulating, deregulating) the role of the private sector in funding and/or delivery of health

---

3   The term "payer" is used of health care in both (social) health insurance systems (the insured) and state/public health care systems (tax payers). In a larger sense, payers can also be purchasers of health services (public or private insurers, social services institutions covering determined population groups), employers contributing to health insurance funds and patients paying out of pocket.

4   Political context: Here we would like to know more about changes affecting health policy competencies (mix/split) at the government level (ministry of health, ministry of labor/social security, ministry of consumer protection, ministry of the environment), shifting competencies and/or responsibilities in the organization of the health care system (funding, remuneration and service delivery). Key words may be: decentralization (devolution, delegation) or centralization trends; role of corporatism and interest group lobbying in health policy making; fragmented levels of responsibility for service delivery (in-patient vs. out-patient services); (changing) role of local government vs. central government in health planning, facility management, etc.; mechanisms of civil society participation in health care issues.

care. Depending on your country, it may be useful to make a distinction between private for-profit and private non-profit health facilities. You may also want to report a development that occurred within the private sector (mergers, concentrations of payers and/or providers, i.e., HMOs/PPOs, health insurances, hospital chains, group practices). However, the invention of a break-through technology should be categorized in the next cluster and not here.

11. New technology:

While we are not interested in all new technologies, this cluster has been included to report and assess technological innovations expected to have a major impact on the effectiveness, quality, costs or the organization of the system (genetic testing, chip card, electronic patient records; teleconsulations, etc.).

12. Others:

If you feel that the health policy development you wish to describe does not fit in any of the clusters, you may create an additional one.

Matrix—Second dimension: Time line/How ideas travel/Process stages

1. Ideas for reform voiced, discussed in different forums (e.g., think tanks, professional/providers' groups, advisory councils, consumer organizations, supranational agencies)—even at an early stage, possibly far from a larger expert audience and/or the political arena
2. Innovations or putting into practice of ideas voiced previously (e.g. at the local level, within institutions, as pilot projects)
3. Acceptance of ideas within relevant professional community and/or (governmental) policy paper at central or regional level
4. Legislative process: This is perhaps the most complex and interesting stage of all, critical for the success or failure of a reform proposal. Please tick here for any legislative proceedings—from the moment a bill is proposed through hearings and lobbying until the effective enactment or rejection of the proposal.
5. Adoption: Measures to facilitate the implementation of a policy at the regulatory and professional level.[5]
6. Evaluation of change—acceptance or failure?
7. Abandonment or further change

---

5 Adoption should include: formulation of accreditation requirements, standards of professional organizations, influence of private sector/market/industry in the adoption process. Note that this step may follow process stage 2 or 3 directly if no legislation was enacted.

The subsequent questions center on the causes and determinants of a particular health policy issue and around the steering and regulatory aspects of this issue.

While we ask you to take into consideration the criteria for the selection of a health policy development (i.e., relevance and scope, impact on status quo, degree of innovation and media coverage/public attention), the choice of what health policy development is worth reporting and commenting on in any given round will obviously depend on your expert judgement.

Please note that the answers to the questions can be brief: Ten to 40 lines per item, or a maximum of three to four pages per policy should do.

We would like to encourage you to structure your responses according to the guiding questions at the beginning of each sub-set, for two reasons: One, the sub-questions under (5) follow the rationale of the time line in the matrix. Two, evaluation and overall reporting will be easier for us when we receive step-by-step answers.

Finally, it would be helpful if you could give references for your information or indicate Web sites for more detailed information on a given policy.

Please photocopy and fill out the following questionnaire for each of the selected health policy issues!

Health Policy Network Questionnaire—Survey # 3
Period covered: October 2003—April 2004

Country: _____

Survey No. _____

Please fill in here the name or names of the authors, co-authors or reviewers who have contributed to this report. If your report is representative of your institution's position, you may want to add the institution's name—e.g., "CRES (review)":

Author/s and/or contributors to this survey: _____

Policy development   #___

1. Title of health policy development reported

_____

Short title

_____

Has this policy been reported in previous surveys?

❏ Yes, in survey # _____, date: _____

❏ No

2. Anchoring the selected health policy issue in the matrix

Please go through the categories of health policy issues listed in the matrix below and tick where appropriate:
- This may be a mark in one box only or a horizontal line if a health policy development has progressed through several columns (stages) during the six months.
- If a policy clearly relates to more than one category (e. g., the introduction of a new remuneration system to facilitate integrated care), then all the appropriate boxes/lines should be marked accordingly.

		Process stages						
	Issue categories	"Idea"[6]	Local or institutional innovation	Acceptance/ Policy paper[7]	Legislative process[8]	Adoption and Implementation[9]	Evaluation	Abandonment/ Change
1.1	Sustainable financing I: Funding and pooling of funds							
1.2	Sustainable financing II: Remuneration/Paying providers							
2	Human resources—training and capacity issues							
3	Quality improvement and assurance							
4	Benefit basket, priority setting							
5	Access to health care (rationing, waiting lists, etc.)							

6	Responsiveness to and empowerment of patients						
7	Political context, e.g. centralized vs. decentralized policy making						
8	Organization/ integration of care across sectors						
9	Long-term care, care for the elderly						
10	Role of private sector						
11	Pharmaceutical policy						
12	New technology						
13	Prevention						
14	Public health						
	Other						

6　This first section refers to any idea floating but not anywhere near a more formal inception stage. Under this heading, you should list ideas that have surfaced only recently and ideas which have been in the pipeline for some time (retrospective view). This means that the reporting period for this column is not restricted to the past six months. That way, we will establish a "stock of health policy ideas-in-development." Over time, we should be able to observe ideas (re)appearing a few years down the road (e.g., medical savings accounts in the Australian health policy debate, Primary Care Trusts in the UK).

7　This refers to any formal written document short of a bill: Tick here for any health policy paper or program, health plan or similar paper issued for the policy described here over the past six months.

8　We renamed this column (previous title: Enactment) to explicitly cover all aspects of the legislative process: from the formal introduction of a bill legislation to parliamentary hearings, lobbying by interest groups and industry and the success (legislation passed) or failure of a proposal.

9　Please use this column for any steps taken towards adoption and implementation at both legal and professional levels: e.g., secondary legislation/regulations, accreditation requirements, organizational standards, etc. That way, the distinction between legislative process and adoption phase should become clear.

3. Content of idea or health policy

Please describe the main objectives, characteristics and expected outcomes of the policy (idea), approach or instrument. What type of incentives (financial, non-financial) are built into or related to this policy? Whom do they affect and how?

_____
_____
_____

Search Results Abstract

This brief abstract will only show on the Web site's search results page when users click on "Show results with summaries." Please describe the purpose and outcome (or expected outcome) of the policy or development you describe in a comprehensive manner (500 characters max.).

_____
_____
_____

Structured summary Q 3 (optional)

Main objectives/characteristics of instrument:

_____
_____
_____

Type of incentives (financial, non-financial):

_____
_____
_____

Group(s) affected
1) _____
2) _____
3) _____
etc.

Sources of information

Please indicate links, papers or publications as suggestions for further reading, as well as the sources of information or data used for this survey.

_____

_____

_____

_____

4. Overall political and economic background of policy development

Was there a change in Government or political direction? Was there a need or pressure to comply with EU legislation (if applicable) or with WTO/GATS regulations?

Has this health policy been derived from or does it aim at attaining a goal formulated in an overall national (or regional) health policy statement such as health policy program, health plan, health goals? If so, which one?

Structured summary Q 4 (optional)

❏ Change of government—comment: _____

❏ Need to comply with EU regulation—comment: _____

❏ Need to comply with WTO/GATS—comment: _____

❏ Need to comply with something else—comment: _____

❏ Change based on an overall national health policy statement (title):

_____

5. Process

5.1 Origins of health policy idea

Where, when, and by whom was the idea generated? What is the main purpose of the health policy idea? What ideas will be used to achieve the idea's or policy's main principle purpose? Who were or are the driving forces behind this idea and why?[10] Is it an entirely new approach, does it follow earlier discussions, has it been borrowed from elsewhere? Is it aimed at amending/updating a prior enactment ("reforming the reform"), and why would it have been passed? Who were the main actors? Are there small-scale examples for this innovation (e.g., at local level, within a single institution, as pilot projects)?

_____

_____

_____

_____

Structured summary Q 5.1 (optional)

Please check, using the text field to specify.

Initiators of idea/main actors

❒ Government/Ministry/Department/Region/Municipality _____
❒ Parliament _____
❒ Providers _____
❒ Payers: insurance company/sickness fund _____
❒ Patients, consumers, etc. _____
❒ Civil society (unions, churches, charities, NGOs, minorities, professional groups, foundations) _____
❒ Scientific community (academic institution, think tank) _____
❒ Private sector or industry _____

---

10 Driving forces/causes could be: Failure or poor performance of a previous approach (which one?), pressure by interest groups (which one[s]?), socio-economic conditions, budget constraints or the media. Also, new ideas may have been initially developed from within single institutions (bottom-up initiatives rather than top-down policy initiatives or legislative motions).

❏ International organizations _____
❏ Media _____
❏ Individual opinion leaders _____
❏ Other driving forces pushing the idea or innovation (please describe):

_____

Approach of idea

The approach of the idea is best described as:

❏ New

❏ Renewed (First voiced, approx. year of entering debate, country of origin?)

_____

❏ An amendment (Of which reform/bill/legislation?)

_____

5.1.3 Innovation or model project

Are there any (small-scale) examples of innovation (experiences)?

❏ No

❏ Yes,
    at the local or regional level: _____
    within institutions: _____
    as a pilot project: _____
    other: _____

5.2 Policy papers and stakeholder positions

How were or are other stakeholders/affected groups positioned towards this idea or policy and its main purpose? Who opposes/opposed this idea or policy and why? Has the idea or policy been accepted by relevant actors; or was it abandoned? Was a policy paper formulated? By whom? Who held the leadership role in bringing forward this idea or policy? Were there alliances between stakeholders in support of the idea or new policy? Who mediated conflicts of interest between stakeholders?

_____

_____

_____

_____

Structured summary Q 5.2 (optional)

Actors: Position toward policy

In the following table, please indicate the position of the major players toward the policy described. For groups or actors not positioned yet or not holding any stakes in the process, do not mark any box. The middle box should be used for neutral actors or those having voiced mixed reactions. In case of the latter, please give details in the space provided above.

A word of caution: A table can only illustrate positions, influences or priorities to some extent. It is not a tool for the analysis of alliances or more complex interaction. For more detailed descriptions, in-depth analysis and/or expert estimates (e.g. concerning the likeliness of success of a health policy or idea, chances of implementation, interest group alliances, etc.) please use the space provided above.

Stakeholder position toward development of idea or policy:

Actor/Position	very strong	strong	neutral	weak	none
Government	☐	☐	☐	☐	☐
Parliament	☐	☐	☐	☐	☐
Providers	☐	☐	☐	☐	☐
Payers	☐	☐	☐	☐	☐

Patients	☐	☐	☐	☐	☐
Civil society	☐	☐	☐	☐	☐
Private sector/ industry (specify)	☐	☐	☐	☐	☐
Scientific community	☐	☐	☐	☐	☐
International organizations	☐	☐	☐	☐	☐
Media	☐	☐	☐	☐	☐
Individual opinion leaders (specify)	☐	☐	☐	☐	☐
Others (specify)	☐	☐	☐	☐	☐

5.3 Legislative process: Influences in policy making and legislation

Did or will the development of this idea or health policy lead to a formal piece of legislation? In how far has the original proposal been changed or modified in the process? Can you describe the powers and the influences of the various actors and stakeholders involved in the legislative process?

_____

_____

_____

_____

Structured summary Q 5.3 (optional)

Legislative process: Outcome

☐ Success
☐ Failure
☐ Major changes
☐ N/A

Actor/Position	very strong	strong	neutral	weak	none
Government	☐	☐	☐	☐	☐
Parliament	☐	☐	☐	☐	☐
Providers	☐	☐	☐	☐	☐
Payers	☐	☐	☐	☐	☐
Patients	☐	☐	☐	☐	☐
Civil society	☐	☐	☐	☐	☐
Private sector/industry (specify)	☐	☐	☐	☐	☐
Scientific community	☐	☐	☐	☐	☐
International organizations	☐	☐	☐	☐	☐
Media	☐	☐	☐	☐	☐
Individual opinion leaders (specify)	☐	☐	☐	☐	☐
Others (specify)	☐	☐	☐	☐	☐

5.4 Adoption and implementation

Which actors and stakeholders were, are or will be involved in the adoption process towards implementation? Which means are necessary, i.e., tools for successful implementation/achievement of policy purpose? Who moderates the process? Were or are these actors and stakeholders actively participating in the process? If not, why? Who else is or will be directly or indirectly affected by implementation? Why and how? How successful was implementation or what are the chances of implementation? (For expert opinion, please use questions 6 and 7.) Where were or are the obstacles? What incentives would facilitate the implementation of this policy, in addition to, or instead of the incentives provided? What was done to convince, or promised to appease, the opponents to this policy?

Structured summary Q 5.4 (optional)

Actors: Priority of policy on their agenda

Actor/Position	very high on agenda	high	neutral	low on agenda	not on agenda
Government	☐	☐	☐	☐	☐
Parliament	☐	☐	☐	☐	☐
Providers	☐	☐	☐	☐	☐
Payers	☐	☐	☐	☐	☐
Patients	☐	☐	☐	☐	☐
Civil society	☐	☐	☐	☐	☐
Private sector/industry (specify)	☐	☐	☐	☐	☐
Scientific community	☐	☐	☐	☐	☐
International organizations	☐	☐	☐	☐	☐
Media	☐	☐	☐	☐	☐
Individual opinion leaders (specify)	☐	☐	☐	☐	☐
Others (specify)	☐	☐	☐	☐	☐

5.5 Monitoring and evaluation

Does this policy foresee a mechanism for regularly reviewing the implementation process, the impact, the overall appropriateness of its objectives and its consistency with your national health policy (where applicable)? If yes, please elaborate. Have precautions been taken to minimize the undesirable effects of the reform? If evaluation has already taken place, please provide results. Did evaluation lead to change or abandonment?

_____

_____

_____

_____

Structured summary Q 5.5 (optional):

Review mechanism

❏ Mid-term review or evaluation

❏ Final evaluation:
    ❏ Internal (e.g., quality management system, quality manager)
    ❏ External (e.g., consulting company, academic institution, independent expert)

Dimension of evaluation

❏ Structure
❏ Process
❏ Outcome

Results? Please describe:

_____

6. Expected outcome/overall assessment of policy (expert opinion)

Looking at the intended objectives and effects of the health policy assessed: Will the policy achieve its objectives? What might be its unexpected or undesirable effects? What are or will be the effects on costs, quality, access/equity etc.?

_____
_____
_____
_____

7. Rating this policy (expert opinion)

7.1 Characteristics of this policy

1. How innovative is the policy in your country's present situation?	☐ traditional approach	☐	☐	☐	☐ innovative approach
2. Was/is the policy process compara-tively ...	☐ consensual	☐	☐	☐	☐ highly controversial
3. Actual or expect-ed impact on status quo	☐ marginal	☐	☐	☐	☐ fundamental
4. Visibility in public discussion (media coverage)	☐ very low	☐	☐	☐	☐ very high
5. Transferability	☐ strongly system/ context-dependent	☐	☐	☐	☐ transferable system-neutral

Please give your overall assessment of this policy.

_____

_____

_____

7.2 Rating the impact of this policy (expert opinion):

6. Impact on quality of health care services	☐ marginal	☐	☐	☐	☐ fundamental
7. Impact on level of equity (access)	☐ system less equitable	☐	☐	☐	☐ system equitable
8. Impact on cost-efficiency	☐ very low	☐	☐	☐	☐ very high

Please comment upon your assessment of the *impact* of this policy:

_____

_____

_____

_____

Thank you for your cooperation!

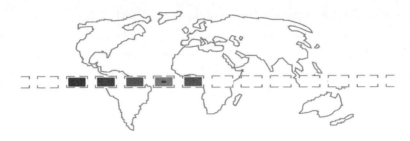

Call for Support

International Network for Health Policy & Reform

Dear friends and colleagues,

With this letter, we cordially invite you to actively support our network. Your contribution of connections, expertise or funding can help us consolidate and broaden our initiative and sustain the continuity of this project through the years to come. Why do we invite you to join us? What's in it for you?

The Bertelsmann Foundation initiated this network of health policy experts to bridge the gap between research and policy. Our reports highlight information— mostly from the world of health economics or medicine—that deserves a broader audience, a wider context. We focus on the politics of policy: the dynamics, interactions and driving forces that bring about health policy reform. If we know the solutions (e.g., evidence-based practice), where do obstacles arise? What makes it so difficult to put sound proposals into effect? The answer to these questions underpins our work. Health policy reform is about interests, values, opportunistic considerations—not just about efficiency, equity, factual evidence or rational decision-making.

So how does health policy work, and why? What can we learn from other countries? Are health reform policies transferable? If so, under what conditions? What constitutes "good" health policy reform? How do various countries cope with demographic transition and technology on the one hand and issues of equity, access and distribution on the other?

Do these questions appeal to you? Join us! You can help us find answers that promote sustainable health policy reform. Are you interested in going beyond what you read in the newspapers or see on television? Join us! You can help us deepen and broaden our network, making it more representative of the health policy reform processes taking place in industrialized countries around the world.

What you can do

You can provide the Health Policy Network with virtual, practical and financial support through one or more of the following activities:
- Become an ambassador
- Become a country patron
- Become a host
- Become a health policy facilitator
- Become a co-publisher
- Become a virtual friend
- Become a peer

Become an ambassador

Inform people, networks and institutions about the International Network for Health Policy & Reform. You can also provide us with names and addresses of representatives (presidents, general secretaries, editors in chief, etc.) in electronic format.

Provide us with member lists (mailing lists, lists of press contacts for scientific journals) so we can inform them about the International Network for Health Policy & Reform, its publications and key findings on an up-to-date basis.

Become a country patron

This form of support allows you to express your particular interest in one or more of the countries in our network. You can also choose to help us add an additional country to the network; we are eager to include any countries with significant, valuable reform experiences to share.

➤ Please contact us to discuss the options and the criteria for inclusion of a country and an appropriate partner institution.

Become a host

As a host, you express your commitment to the network at its liveliest: Your generous grant funds the network's annual meeting, which takes place in a different location each year, in early July or early September.

Your sponsorship of a network meeting covers accommodations and catering for the network experts, special guests and key speakers, for two days (three nights).

In July 2004, we will hold our third meeting in Berlin, Germany. The venue will be the Bertelsmann Company's new conference center right in the heart of the city.

Our fourth meeting, near Barcelona, Spain, is conveniently scheduled to allow our experts to attend the iHEA Biannual Conference in July 2005.

Become a health policy facilitator

Health policy facilitators enable bi-, tri- or multilateral exchange on specific areas of health policy reform. In a closed working setting, our practice-oriented technical briefings bring together the thinkers and the doers from science and practice, philosophy and politics, to look into experiences, investigate transferability, and jointly develop applicable solutions to shared problems.

Topics could be

- Integrated care and disease management programs for chronic disease: getting incentives right (a detailed workshop outline for an expert meeting in October 2004 is available upon request)
- Coping with the workforce gap in nursing
- Wellness in old age: strategies toward healthy aging
- The role of commissions, lobbyists, and scientists in health policy reform: How much advice (science) does the government really need?
- Communication in health policy reform: Can economists talk to lawmakers?
- Ethics and health finance: Is transparency the solution when tradeoffs are tough?